The Family Gi Diet

Rick Gallop and Dr Ruth Gallop

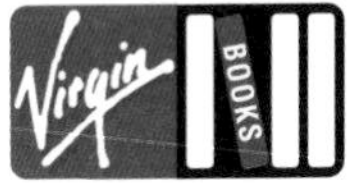

ACKNOWLEDGEMENTS

My thanks go to the readers of the Gi Diet as they have been the inspiration for this book. I have received thousands of emails expressing interest or concern over managing the family's nutrition and health. As most of the writers were women, we have endeavoured to address these issues through their eyes. Nutrition and health truly are a family affair.

On a more personal note, I would like to thank Carolyn Thorne and Gareth Fletcher at Virgin Books for their patience and support throughout the complex process of bringing this book into print.

This edition first published in Great Britain in 2006 by:
Virgin Books Ltd
Thames Wharf Studios
Rainville Road
London
W6 9HA

Published by arrangement with Random House Canada, a division of Random House of Canada Limited

A catalogue record for this book is available from the British Library.

ISBN: 0 7535 0918 0

The paper used in this book is a natural, recyclable product made from wood grown in sustainable forests. The manufacturing process conforms to the regulations of the country of origin.

Designed by Oh Paxton

Printed and bound in Great Britain

Contents

To our sons: Michael, Stephen and David for their joyful tolerance and enthusiastic involvement in Dad's family food experiments over the years.

Foreword

You've got to start somewhere, but there's no point starting a diet unless you intend to be successful. That's what this book is all about: helping you succeed in reaching your goal of a much healthier lifestyle, not just in the short term but from now on. And it's not just for you but for your entire family.

What's so special about this diet book? Why follow its advice rather than the suggestions found in all the other diet books on the shelf? The Gi Diet is nutritionally sound and scientifically based. It takes complex nutritional concepts and makes them easy to understand and put into practice with a creative traffic light system. The Gi Diet offers no gimmicks or quick fixes. It is sustainable. It is transforming.

This book, *The Family Gi Diet*, takes the proven, best-selling concepts of the original *Gi Diet* one important step further: it addresses the entire family. It allows spouses to support one another in the difficult tasks of weight control and eating properly. It deals with age and gender differences. It encourages parents to serve as role models for their children. It makes parents aware of the various behavioural stages of childhood that must be appreciated to improve that most basic of activities, the family meal.

The author, Rick Gallop, is a very special person. He is bright, articulate and innovative. Rick's credentials for writing a diet book are a bit unusual. He is not a nutritionist, nor is he a physician. But for 15 years, he served as president of the Heart and Stroke Foundation of Ontario. He developed a passion for promoting healthy lifestyles that reduce the risk of cardiovascular disease and its devastating consequences. Rick became frustrated at the high failure rates associated with most diet plans. So, true to his character, he sought to devise a better diet method. And he did.

Ultimately, improving how you and your loved ones live is up to you. If you need some help with this, *The Family Gi Diet* is a wonderful guide that will make your entire family feel better and stay healthier. Enjoy the book and enjoy each other.

Norman R. Saunders, MD, FRCP(C)
Department of Pediatrics
University of Toronto

What is special about being a family doctor is having the chance to accompany a family through many of life's stages. Where else in medicine does one get to witness children progressing from birth to adolescence and on to adulthood, or middle-aged patients moving on to grapple with retirement or deteriorating health? I have been practising for over 20 years, and the infants I once cared for are now expecting their own children, the young mothers whom I once commiserated with about their sleepless nights are now losing sleep because of hot flushes. As time has passed I have also witnessed the impact of information technology, which has transformed passive patients into active health-care advocates who are interested in maintaining health and preventing illness.

At any life stage, nutrition is a primary concern. For this reason, I have welcomed the Gi Diet as an excellent resource when counselling patients. Diets in general have been anathema to me, because by their very nature they have a start point and an end point, with consequent rebounding and accumulation of even more weight. The Gi approach is more of a lifestyle than a diet, and it is sustainable because it is based on sound scientific principles. Organising foods in categories based on the colours of a traffic light provides a straightforward system of eating that anyone can grasp and apply.

In *The Family Gi Diet*, Rick Gallop takes the programme further by recommending practices to last a lifetime. There is excellent advice on including children in grocery shopping and meal preparation, plus setting clear but flexible limits regarding mealtimes and snacks. One significant piece of information they share is that it takes 10–15 exposures to a new food for a child to accept it. This means parents should not give up introducing their children to vegetables if they initially refuse them. The book also emphasises the importance of exercise, especially for seniors. This advice is supported by the World Health Organisation's preliminary findings that eating well and exercising not only extend one's lifespan but also prevent infirmity.

The Gi Diet is a weight-loss programme that I am able to endorse as I see its results with my own eyes. Patients thank me for recommending the diet to them because they've lost weight and feel more energetic than ever. Embarking on this programme has immediate health benefits and also teaches us life lessons about staying well.

Pauline Pariser, MAsc, MD, CCFP, CFCP
Assistant Professor
Department of Family and Community Medicine
University of Toronto

Introduction

My first book, *The Gi Diet*, was published in 2002 and quickly became one of the most successful diet books ever, with more than 1.5 million copies sold. It is currently available in 15 countries worldwide, in a dozen different languages. But my greatest delight has been the enormous number of readers' emails I've received. I had no idea that the book would generate such a flood of responses, and I was amazed to hear about all the ways in which this new approach to eating has actually changed people's lives. I've heard from tens of thousands of readers, in messages that are personal, thoughtful, supportive – and frequently ecstatic!

It was this feedback that encouraged me to embark on this new book, *The Family Gi Diet*. Why focus on the family? The first reason is that most of the correspondence I've received has been from women. And despite all the changes in family life, for better or worse most women still play the role of chief shopper, cook and gatekeeper for their family's health and nutrition. At the same time, women, as well as men, are working longer hours outside the house. They just can't devote a lot of their time to 'managing' the way the family eats. One of their biggest challenges is how to prepare a different set of diet meals for themselves while cooking for the rest of the family. How can they control their own weight, meet the needs and culinary whims of the rest of the family and somehow avoid becoming a short-order cook?

There's another consideration as well. Men and women have different nutritional needs, depending on their stage of life and hormonal factors. A woman expecting twins won't have the same appetite and nutritional demands as the elderly grandfather who might be sharing the dinner table with her.

Menopause also brings its own metabolic changes and nutritional shifts for women. And teenagers may have a strange concept of what constitutes a 'hearty breakfast'. My wife, Ruth, and I have raised three children – one of them a vegetarian – so we're well aware of the challenges of feeding a family whose members' appetites and tastes vary.

Women are not only concerned about their own weight, but they also worry about their overweight spouses, partners and children. Is your partner overweight? Since over 60% of men in the UK are either in that category or officially obese, there is a good chance that this is the case. (See the Body Mass Index on page 30 to see if he qualifies.)

And you've probably been reading about the alarming increase in childhood obesity. According to recent studies, the number of obese children between six and fifteen years old has trebled in the last decade. At the same time, you don't want your children – especially your daughters – to become obsessed with weight loss and body image. What you *do* want is to establish healthy patterns of eating that keep your children fit and energetic, not only as they are growing up but for the rest of their lives. What you *don't* want to do is cater to their every whim by cooking three different meals every night. You can't really blame kids for their cravings. With so many processed, over-advertised, high-fat snack foods available, they are simply following the path of least resistance. We need to give them appealing options.

So I could see that a family approach to the Gi Diet would be helpful, and the result is this book, *The Family Gi Diet*. I persuaded my wife Ruth, who is Professor Emeritus of the Faculties of Nursing and Medicine at the University of Toronto, to provide a female perspective, as well as to share her experience in women's health issues and behavioural research. She wrote Chapter 7, which outlines the special nutritional needs of women from menarche to menopause and beyond, and gave valuable information on feeding children at various stages of their life. Together we talk about how to follow the Gi Diet along with spouses, partners, toddlers and teenagers. We give you help with shopping, meal planning and lunch packing, and have included 50 new delicious recipes that are Gi versions of family favourites. We address the special needs of seniors, who are often neglected in other diet books, and help you use nutrition to reduce your family's risk of heart disease, stroke, diabetes, most cancers and even degenerative conditions like Alzheimer's. The evidence from medical research is overwhelming that weight management and diet are the most effective ways to reduce your risk of these life-threatening diseases. So the Gi Diet is not just about losing weight simply and painlessly; it's also about a permanent gain in quality of life.

On the Gi Diet, you won't go hungry or feel deprived, and you will never have to count another calorie or carb. I'm a firm believer that a diet shouldn't have to involve higher maths! How is this possible? The keys are simplicity and nutritional balance. With its emphasis on fruits, vegetables, whole grains, low-fat dairy products, lean meat and seafood, the Gi Diet is an ideal way for the whole family to eat, whether weight control is an issue or not. And if you or your partner needs to shed 5 pounds or 50, *The Family Gi Diet* will show both of you how to eat more healthily and lose weight from the same menu.

For more information on the Gi Diet, a free subscription to my quarterly newsletter, and details about how to contact me, visit **www.gidiet.com**. I would love to hear from you.

The Gi Diet Programme

1 Why do you want to lose weight?

Do you want to lose 10 pounds or 100? Perhaps you just want to drop a dress size or two while you help your overweight partner lose a significant amount of weight. It's important to look at the reasons why you or members of your family want to lose weight; your answer will have a lot to do with your motivation to start and, more important, to stay the course with your new way of eating.

Let's look at the most common reasons why people want to lose weight and see how they reflect your own.

1. I WANT TO LOOK BETTER

Judging from the correspondence I have received – 20,000 emails and counting – the day when people discover that they have to dig out their 'skinny' pants again is at least as rewarding as seeing the numbers fall on the scale. Most of us would rather shop for clothes that flatter and show off the body rather than resort to camouflage. It's a powerful motivator to walk into a room and hear a friend ask, 'Have you lost weight? You look terrific.' I've sold more books based on word of mouth – people asking *Gi Diet* readers how they lost their weight – than through any other marketing strategy.

But losing weight is not just about trying to live up to unreachable, red-carpet standards of beauty or thinness; it's about feeling at ease in your body and liking what you see in the mirror. Weight loss boosts self-esteem and confidence, for women in particular, which in turn makes it easier to maintain new eating habits. It's amazing the difference the loss of just a few pounds can make, not only to how you look in your clothes but to how you feel about yourself.

Dear Rick
I lost 6 stone in 22 weeks, but the real news is what a difference the weight change has made to my appearance. I went to a family wedding last week and was embarrassed by the attention I got. The room seemed to stop and gasp when I walked into the reception! I lost count of how many people asked what happened, told me how good I looked, asked what diet I was on and how much weight I had lost. By the way, my cholesterol and other health stats are fantastic! There is certainly no more rewarding personal journey than transforming your body into what you always wanted it to be. I can't begin to express how valuable the Gi Diet has been to making this happen.
Derek

2. I WANT TO FEEL MORE ENERGETIC AND LESS LETHARGIC
Perhaps what I hear about most frequently from readers, other than the thrill of losing pounds or going down a dress size, is the surge of energy that comes with a lighter, healthier body. I witnessed a dramatic demonstration of the kind of burden extra weight can be just the other day. My wife and I had just completed some house renovations to suit our empty-nest lifestyle, and as we were restoring some order, I asked Ruth to carry a couple of 20-pound dumb-bells up a flight of stairs to my new workout room. She could only get them to the first floor landing before she had to put them down again. 'How do people who are 40 pounds overweight get around, let alone climb stairs?' she wondered. And 40 pounds of extra weight is not something you can just put down when you want to. Imagine

the energy that goes into carrying those pounds! That's the energy that will be available to you again if you shed the excess weight.

Readers also tell me about the delight they experience when they find themselves able to do more exercise and to enjoy activities they haven't participated in since their teens. If regaining your former energy and vitality is important to you, you'll receive constant motivation as your new, lighter body rejoices in its recently acquired freedom to run, swim, play squash, or engage in any activity you may have given up for 'lack of energy'.

3. I WANT TO BE HEALTHIER, AND I WANT TO HELP MY FAMILY BECOME HEALTHIER

Although health may not be your primary reason for losing weight, it is ultimately the most important one. Excess weight and poor diet are by far the most critical factors in increasing your chances of developing major diseases that can either undermine your quality of life or drastically shorten it. These include heart disease, stroke, cancer, diabetes and Alzheimer's. Of course, genes play a role in your risk of these diseases too, but anyone who is overweight and undernourished is putting him or herself at risk for these conditions. The prospect of a long life, especially one free of pain, disability and disease, is a powerful motivator.

Keeping in mind these three incentives – looking and feeling better, enjoying greater energy and improving your overall health – will go a long way in helping you stick to the Gi Diet and will open up a whole new chapter in your life. But if losing weight has so many obvious benefits, why is the prevalence of overweight and obesity steadily increasing, especially as hundreds of new diet books flood the stores each year? Well, the fact is that most diets don't work. And the reason they fail is that people don't stay on them. Why do they give up? I'm sure the following explanations will be familiar to you.

WHY DIETS DON'T WORK

- Most diets leave you feeling hungry, weak and deprived. You stagger through the day with a grumbling stomach, but sooner or later you cave in and order a pizza with double cheese. Feeling perpetually hungry is the primary reason that people give up on their diet.
- The diet is too complicated and time-consuming to follow. You spend each day weighing and measuring food, calculating carbs or calories and keeping food diaries. Perhaps this is fun initially, but then it all just becomes a burden. You're too busy to follow a diet that feels more like a maths exam.
- You feel bad. Many diets cut out essential nutrients, leaving you feeling lethargic, lacking energy and concerned about your health. Is it little wonder people give up?

WHY HAVE WE BECOME SO FAT?

Around 43% of men and 33% of women in the UK are overweight, and an additional 22% of men and 23% of women are obese. In the last decade the percentage of adults who are obese has increased by over 50%. The rate of increase in obesity in children is even worse. So what's happening to us? Why, in a relatively short time, have we gained so much weight?

It's not as if we lack awareness of weight issues. There are shelves of books and racks of magazines with cover stories on diets and fitness regimens. The media have latched onto the 'obesity epidemic' with a fervour – fat is big news these days.

The answer to our collective weight crisis is simple: we're consuming more calories than we're expending, and the resulting surplus is stored around our waists, hips and thighs as fat. (Maybe it's found a nice spot on your upper arms, too.) There's no mystery here. But to understand why we seem to be consuming more calories, we need to get back to basics and look at the three fundamental elements of our diet: carbohydrates, fats and proteins. I'm sure you've heard about these characters. We need to understand how they work together, whether we're in the process of getting fat or thin, and the role they play in our digestive system.

We'll start with protein, since the popularity of high-protein diets like the Atkins programme has made it a hot topic.

PROTEIN

Protein is an essential part of your diet. In fact, you are already half protein: 50% of your dry body weight is made up of muscles, organs, skin and hair, all forms of protein. We need this element to build and repair body tissues, and it figures in nearly all metabolic reactions. Protein is also a critical brain food, providing amino acids for the neurotransmitters that relay messages to the brain. The brain fog people experience on some diets, therefore, is probably the result of diminished protein. This is also why it's not a good idea to skip breakfast on the morning of a big meeting or exam. Protein is literally food for thought.

The main sources of dietary protein come from animals: meat, seafood, dairy and eggs. Vegetable sources include beans and soy-based products like tofu. Unfortunately, protein sources such as red meat and full-fat dairy products are also high in saturated fats (see page 13), which are harmful to your health, especially your heart. This is why there is so much concern in the medical field about the popularity of high-protein/low-carb diets like Atkins. The problem is not so much with the high levels of protein, but with the saturated fats associated with these proteins.

It is important that we get our protein from sources that are low in saturated fats, such as lean meats, skinless poultry, seafood, low-fat dairy products and tofu and other soy products. One exceptional source of protein is the humble bean. Beans are just about a perfect food – they're high in protein and fibre, and low in saturated fat. No wonder so many of the world's cuisines have found myriad wonderful ways to cook beans. We need to become more bean savvy. Nuts are another excellent source of protein that are relatively low in fat – as long as you don't eat a whole bowlful.

In terms of how you feel, protein is what leaves you feeling satisfied and well fed. Because it breaks down more slowly in your digestive system, you feel fuller longer. This characteristic is key to the success of the Gi Diet.

Now let's consider that most maligned and misunderstood food group: fats.

FATS

Low-fat is good; no-fat is not an option. Fats are essential for the digestive process, cell development and overall health. Despite their bad reputation, they are as essential as protein to your overall diet.

Oddly enough, fats aren't necessarily what make you fat. It's the *quantity* of fat you consume that makes the difference; fat has more than twice the calories per gram than either carbohydrates or proteins. So if you decide to 'just add peanut butter' to your otherwise disciplined regime, it doesn't take much of it – two tablespoons – to spike your total calorie count.

Also, once you eat fat, your body is a genius at hanging onto it and refusing to let it go. This is because fat is how the body stores reserve supplies of energy, usually around the waist, hips and thighs. Fat is money in the bank as far as the body is concerned – a rainy-day investment for when you have to call up extra energy. This clever system originally helped our ancestors survive during periods of famine. The problem today is that we don't live with cycles of feast and famine – it's more like feast, and then feast again! But the body's eagerness for fat continues, along with its reluctance to give it up.

This is why losing weight is so difficult: your body does everything it can to persuade you to eat more fat! How? Through fat's capacity to make things taste good. So it's not just you who thinks that juicy steaks, chocolate cake and rich ice cream taste better than a bean sprout. That's the fat content of cake and steak talking.

Sorry to say, there's no getting around it: if you want to lose weight, you have to watch your fat consumption. In addition, you need to be concerned about the *type* of fat you eat. Although this has no effect on weight, it definitely has an impact on our health. Your risk of heart disease, stroke, colon and other cancers, and Alzheimer's is significantly influenced by the type of fat in your diet. So here's the skinny on fat.

Fat comes in four varieties: the best, which actually benefits your health, the good, the bad and the really ugly. Let's start with the nasty one.

The 'really ugly' fats are potentially the most dangerous, and they lurk in many of the most popular snack foods. They are the **trans fats** you've been hearing about – vegetable oils that have been heat treated to make them thicken. These hydrogenated oils, or trans fatty acids, take on the worst characteristics of saturated fats (see below), so don't use them at all. And avoid packaged snack foods, baked goods, crackers and cereals that contain them. (You can spot them by checking the label for 'hydrogenated' or 'partly hydrogenated' oils.)

The 'bad' fats are called **saturated fats**. They are the more familiar form, and they almost always come from animal sources. These are the fats that solidify at room temperature. Butter, cheese, hard 'stick' margarine and many meats are all high in saturated fats. But there are a couple of other sources of saturated fats you should be aware of: coconut oil and palm oil are the only vegetable oils that are saturated, and because they are cheap, you will find them used in many snack foods, especially cookies. These saturated fats elevate your risk of the life-threatening diseases we mentioned earlier. The evidence is also growing that many cancers, including colon, prostate and breast, are associated with diets high in saturated fats.

The 'good' fats are the **polyunsaturated fats**, and they are cholesterol-free. Most vegetable oils, such as corn and sunflower, fall into this category. But they're still fat, and they still pack calories.

What you really *should* be eating, however, are the **monounsaturated fats**, which actually promote good health. These are the fats found in olives, almonds, and rapeseed and olive oils. Monounsaturated fats have a beneficial effect on cholesterol and help protect your heart. This is one reason why the incidence of heart disease is low in Mediterranean countries, where olive oil is a staple. Although fancy olive oil is expensive, you can enjoy the same health benefits from less costly supermarket brands. It doesn't have to be extra-virgin, double cold pressed.

Another highly beneficial oil that falls into its own category is **omega-3**, a fatty acid that is found in deep-sea fish, such as salmon, mackerel, tuna and herring, as well as in lake trout, walnuts, and flaxseed and rapeseed oils. Some brands of eggs also contain omega-3 oils, which can help lower cholesterol and protect your cardiovascular health.

Even though more of us are buying low-fat foods and drinking more low-fat milk, our overall consumption of fat remains stubbornly consistent. Why? It's partly the result of a big increase in cheese and ice cream consumption, as well as the 'silent' fats that are hidden in some of our favourite foods, such as crackers, muffins, cereals and fast foods. A McDonald's Grilled Veggie Melt may sound like a healthier choice, but it still contains 21 grams of fat. So even though fat consumption has not changed significantly over the past decade, the percentage of overweight people in the population has soared. We can't pin that on fat consumption alone, however. What has increased is our consumption of grain. Since grain is a carbohydrate, let's look at this third component of our diet, and whether carbs deserve their bad rap.

CARBOHYDRATES

Carbohydrates are the primary source of energy for our bodies, and they usually account for more than 50% of our diet. They've been so much in the news over the past few years that a new word has entered the language: 'carbs'. They are found, for instance, in grains, vegetables, fruits, legumes (beans), pasta and dairy products. (They're in cheesecake too, but that's another matter.)

Here is how carbs work: when you eat a mango, your body digests the carbohydrates in the fruit and turns them into glucose, which provides us with energy. The glucose dissolves in your bloodstream and then travels to the parts of your body that use energy, such as your muscles and brain. This is why a high-carb treat like a Danish starts to beckon in mid-afternoon, when your energy flags, but as you will soon understand, it is selecting the right type of carb that will help you achieve your optimum energy and weight. So carbohydrates are critical to everyone's health. They are also rich in fibre, vitamins and minerals, including antioxidants, which we now know play an important role in the prevention of heart disease and cancer.

Most of our carbs come from grains – from breads, cereals, bagels, pasta, crackers and innocent snacks like Melba toast, as well as from double-fudge cookies. And we're eating more and more of these foods; over the past three decades, our consumption of grains has increased by 50%. That fact is alarming enough, but the *quality* of the grain we eat has changed, too. A little detour into some food history will be helpful here.

Humans began cultivating grain only 10,000 years ago. That seems like a long time, but from an evolutionary standpoint, it's a mere blink of an eye. The fertile lands of Egypt became the breadbasket of the ancient world, providing grain that became the staple food of the West, just as rice was for the East. Grain was made into flour by grinding stones driven by wind or water. Coarse-ground whole grains became the foundation of our diet for thousands of years.

Then, only a few generations ago, everything changed with the Agrarian Revolution. New technology made refrigeration and mass production of food possible. The miller's traditional wind and water mills were replaced by high-speed steel rolling mills, which stripped away most of the key nutrients, including fibre and wheat-germ oils (which could spoil), to produce a talcum-like powder: today's white flour. This fine white flour is the basic ingredient for most of our baked goods, breads and cereals, as well as for such snack foods as doughnuts, muffins, tortilla chips, pretzels and cookies. Walk through any supermarket and you will be surrounded by towering stacks of these flour-based processed products.

The days of eating food that came straight from the farmer to the dinner table were over. The food processor, the food packer and those big trucks full of Wonder Bread became the intermediary. All the giant food companies – Kraft, Kellogg's, Del Monte, Nestlé – were born in the 20th century. But with changes in the economy and culture that saw women enter the labour force in increasing numbers, we happily spent more money for the convenience of prepared, processed, packaged, canned, frozen and bottled food. The TV Dinner era had begun.

Unfortunately, our bodies have paid the price for this convenience and the year-round availability of 'fresh' foods. The processing that is required to prevent spoilage has reduced the nutritional value of our food. Processed, low-fibre food also has a direct link to the growing number of cures for constipation in the drugstore aisles. The more food is processed beyond its natural, fibrous state, the less processing your body has to do to digest it. And the quicker you digest food, the sooner you feel hungry again – and so the more you eat. You can test the difference by eating a bowl of sugary cold cereal one morning and a bowl of old-fashioned, slow-cooking oatmeal the next. The oatmeal 'sticks to your ribs' (as my mother used to say), keeping you satisfied all morning, whereas the cold cereal leaves you looking for a muffin by the time you get to the office.

The explanation for our collective weight problem, then, is that we are eating foods that our bodies don't have to work very hard to digest. I'm not going to suggest that we all go back to the land, grow our own grain and haul it off to the local miller. Those days are over. But we need to somehow slow down the digestive process so that we feel hungry less often.

How can we do that? The only practical solution is to eat foods that release their nutrients slowly, so they break down at a slow and steady rate in our digestive system. The result is that we feel fuller for longer periods. This postpones the feeling of hunger, allowing us to eat less food. That's the simple secret to the effectiveness of the Gi Diet. It's hard to believe that weight loss can go hand in hand with a programme that includes three meals and three snacks a day, and leaves you feeling satisfied. You can eat often and well, if you follow the simple programme outlined in the next chapter.

SUMMARY

- Eat carbohydrates that have not been highly processed and that do not contain highly processed ingredients.
- Eat less fat overall and look for low-fat alternatives to your current diet.
- Eat monounsaturated and polyunsaturated fats only.
- Include some protein in all your meals and snacks.
- Eat only low-fat protein, preferably from both animal and vegetable sources.

2 The Gi Diet

The 'Gi' in Gi Diet stands for glycaemic index, which is the basis of this diet (and the only scientific phrase you'll need to know). The glycaemic index is the secret to reducing calories and losing weight without going hungry. It measures the speed at which carbohydrates break down in our digestive system and turn into glucose, the body's source of energy or, put another way, the gas in our body's tank.

The glycaemic index was developed by Dr David Jenkins, professor of nutritional sciences at the University of Toronto, when he was researching the impact of different carbohydrates on the blood sugar or glucose level of people with diabetes. He found that certain carbohydrates broke down quickly and flooded the bloodstream with sugar, but others broke down more slowly, only marginally increasing blood sugar levels. The faster a food breaks down, the higher the rating on the glycaemic index, which sets sugar at 100 and scores all other foods against that number. These findings were important to those people with diabetes, who could then use the index to identify low-Gi, slow-release foods that would help to control their blood sugar levels. Here are some examples of the Gi rating for a range of popular foods:

EXAMPLES OF GI RATINGS

High Gi foods		Low Gi foods	
Sugar	100	Orange	44
Baguette	95	All-Bran	43
Cornflakes	84	Oatmeal	42
Rice cake	82	Spaghetti	41
Doughnut	76	Apple	38
Bagel	72	Beans	31
Cereal bar	72	Grapefruit	25
Biscuit	69	Plain yogurt	14

What do these Gi ratings have to do with the numbers on your bathroom scales? Well, it turns out that low-Gi, slow-release foods have a significant impact on our ability to lose weight. As I have explained, when we eat a high-Gi food, the body quickly digests it and releases a flood of sugar (glucose) into the bloodstream. This gives us a short-term high, but the sugar is just as quickly absorbed by the body, leaving us with that familiar post-sugar slump. We feel lethargic and start looking for our next sugar fix. So a fast-food lunch of a double cheeseburger, coke and fries will deliver a short-term burst of energy, but by mid-afternoon we start feeling tired, sluggish and hungry. That's when we reach for a 'one-time-only' brownie or packet of crisps. These high-Gi foods deliver the rush we want and then let us down again. And so on. The roller coaster is a hard cycle to break. But a high-Gi diet will make you feel hungry more often, and so you end up eating more and gaining more weight.

Let's look at the other end of the Gi index. Low-Gi foods, such as fruits, vegetables, whole grains, pasta, beans and low-fat dairy products take longer to digest, deliver a steady supply of sugar to our bloodstream and leave us feeling fuller for a longer time. Consequently, we eat less. It also helps that these foods are lower in calories, too. As a result, we consume less food and fewer calories, without going hungry or feeling unsatisfied.

INSULIN

The key player in this process of energy storage and retrieval is insulin, a hormone secreted by the pancreas. Insulin does two things very well. First, it regulates the amount of sugar (glucose) in our bloodstream, removing the excess and storing it as glycogen for immediate use by our muscles, or putting it into long-term storage as fat. Second, insulin acts as a security guard at the fat gates, reluctantly giving up its reserves. So fat is easy to acquire and hard to lose. (Or as they say, two minutes on the lips, two months on the hips.)

I was recently on vacation in a remote part of central Mexico, visiting the Copper Canyon, which, incredibly, is larger and deeper than the Grand Canyon in Arizona. A tribe of Tarahumara Indians still resides there. Until recently, these indigenous peoples typically put on 30 pounds during the summer and autumn, when the crops, particularly corn, were plentiful. Then, over the course of the winter, when food became scarce, they lost these 30 pounds. Insulin was the champion in this process, both helping accumulate fat and then guarding its depletion.

Of course, food is now readily available, as close as the nearest 24-hour supermarket. But our bodies still function very much as they did in the earliest days.

Insulin is stimulated when we eat high-Gi foods. The job of insulin is to reduce the sugar levels in our blood, which, if left unchecked, would lead to hyperglycaemia. If we aren't using all that energy at the moment, the glucose is stored as fat. Soon we become hungry again. Our body will either draw on our reserves of fat and laboriously convert them back to sugar or it will look for more food. Giving up extra fat is the body's last choice – who knows when that supply might come in handy! So your body would rather send you to the fridge than work to convert fat back to sugar. This helped serve survival back in the old days, but it gets in the way of weight loss now.

So our goal is to limit the amount of insulin in our system by avoiding high Gi foods and instead choosing low-Gi foods.

This will keep the supply of sugar in our bloodstream consistent. This means we don't feel hungry. That hollow, empty feeling, the one that sooner or later drives a dieter to the fridge, will be headed off at the pass. Slow-release, low-Gi carbohydrates help curb your appetite by leaving you feeling fuller for a longer period of time. When you combine them with lean protein and the best fats which help slow the digestive process, you have the magic combination that will allow you to lose weight without going hungry.

Translated into real food, what does this mean? Well, for dinner you could have a grilled chicken breast (without the skin), boiled new potatoes, a side salad of cos lettuce and red pepper, dressed with a bit of olive oil and lemon, and some asparagus if you feel like it. The trick is to stick to foods that have a low Gi, are low in fat (particularly saturated fat) and low-ish in calories. This sounds – and, in fact, is – quite complex. And it also sounds as if I'm breaking my promise of simplicity. But don't worry: we've done all the calculations, measurements and maths for you, and sorted the foods you like to eat into easy-to-follow, traffic-light colours.

Dear Rick

I began eating the Gi way for almost two months and I'm thrilled with the results I've had so far. I feel so much better and have lost 1 stone. I've combined the Gi Diet with working out for 30 minutes 3 times a week.

As a teacher, I used to feel like I would hit a wall at about 1.30 every afternoon. But now that my blood sugar levels are more consistent, I feel fine throughout the afternoon, and always have a food bar handy in my desk in case I feel a little hungry. I guess the best thing is that I don't feel deprived or that I'm on a diet. Rather, I just feel I'm eating better.

Thanks so much!

Mary

The Gi Diet's emphasis on fruits, vegetables, whole grains, beans and low-fat dairy products, along with lean protein and 'good' fats, is a nutritionally ideal way to eat. In short, the Gi Diet keeps you feeling satisfied and energetic; the traffic-light colour coding means never having to count calories or points, or weigh and measure foods; and, finally, it's highly nutritional and good for your health.

HOW TO FOLLOW THE GI DIET

Now that you have a little grounding in the science of the Gi diet, let's get down to the nitty-gritty: what to eat and what to avoid; how much to eat; how often to eat.

WHAT DO I EAT?

To find out what to eat and what to avoid check out the Complete Gi Diet Food Guide on pages 234-47. Here's how the colour-coded categories work:

- **Red-light foods**: Avoid these. They are the high-Gi, higher-calorie foods.

- **Yellow-light foods**: The foods in the yellow column are mid-range Gi foods and should be treated with caution. There are two phases in the Gi Diet: Phase I is the weight-loss portion of the diet and yellow-light foods should be avoided during this time. Once you've reached your target weight and you enter Phase II, the maintenance phase, you can begin to enjoy yellow-light foods from time to time.
- **Green-light foods**: This column lists foods that are low-Gi, low in fat and lower in calories. These are the foods that will make you lose weight. Don't expect them to be tasteless and boring! There are many delicious and satisfying choices that will make you feel as though you aren't even on a diet.

If you're a veteran of the low-carbohydrate craze, you'll be surprised to find potatoes and rice in the green-light column, but they are fine as long as they the right type. Baked potatoes and French fries have a high Gi, while boiled, small new potatoes have a low Gi. With rice, the short-grain, glutinous variety served in Chinese and Thai restaurants is high-Gi, while long-grain, brown, basmati and wild rice are low. Pasta is also a green-light food – as long as it is cooked only until al dente (with some firmness to the bite). Any processing of food, including cooking, will increase its Gi rating, since heat breaks down a food's starch capsules and fibre, giving your digestive juices a head start. This is why you should never overcook vegetables; instead steam them or boil them in a small amount of water until they are just tender. This way they will retain their vitamins and other nutrients, and their Gi rating will remain low.

Chapter 4 outlines the best green-light options for breakfast, lunch, dinner and snacks.

HOW MUCH DO I EAT?

You can, with a few exceptions (marked with asterisks), eat as much of the green-light foods as you like within reason (five heads of cabbage might be going too far). This isn't a deprivation diet. While following the Gi programme, you should be eating three meals and three snacks daily. Don't leave your digestive system with nothing to do. The saying 'The devil finds work for idle hands' might also be applied to your stomach. If your digestive system is busy processing food and steadily supplying energy to your brain, you won't be looking for high-calorie snacks.

Recommended Green-Light Servings	
Green-light breads (these have at least 2 1/2–3g of fibre per slice)	1 slice
Green-light cereals	120g (4oz)
Green-light nuts	8–10
Margarine (non-hydrogenated, light)	2 tsp
Meat, fish, poultry	120g (4oz) (about the size of a pack of cards)
Olive/rapeseed oil	1 tsp
Olives	4–5
Pasta	40g (1 1/2 oz) uncooked
Potatoes (new, boiled)	2–3
Rice (basmati, brown, long-grain)	50g (1 3/4oz) uncooked

Phase II	
Chocolate (at least 70% cocoa)	2 squares
Red wine	1 glass (125 ml/5 fl oz)

Portions

Each meal and snack should contain, if possible, a combination of green-light protein, carbohydrates – especially fruit and vegetables – and fats. An easy way to visualise what size these portions should be is to imagine your plate divided into three sections. Half the plate should be covered with vegetables; one quarter should contain protein, such as lean meats, seafood, eggs or, if vegetarian, tofu or soy-based foods; and the last quarter should contain a green-light serving of rice, pasta or potatoes.

Here is how your Gi Diet green-light plate should look:

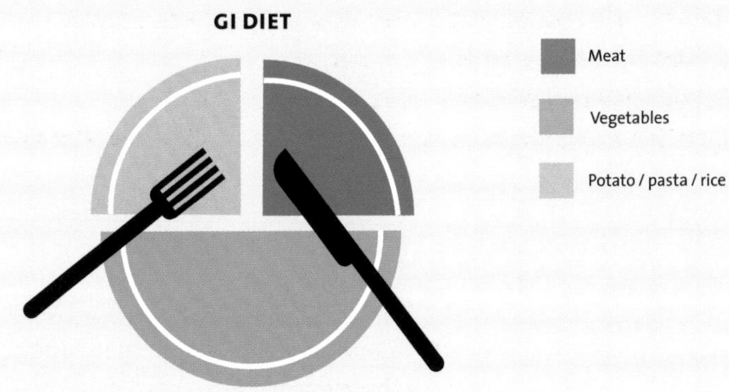

WHEN DO I EAT?

Try to eat regularly throughout the day. If you skimp on breakfast and lunch, you will probably be starving by dinner and pile on the food then. Have one snack mid-morning, another mid-afternoon and one before bed. The idea is to keep your digestive system happily busy so you won't start craving those red-light snacks.

Now that you know how the Gi Diet works it's time to get started. In the next chapter we've outlined the steps for beginning Phase 1.

Note: Before starting any major change in your eating patterns, make sure you check with your doctor.

SUMMARY

1. Low Gi foods are slower to digest, so you feel satisfied longer.
2. The key to losing weight is to eat low Gi, low calorie foods.
3. In Phase I, eat only green-light foods.
4. Eat three balanced meals and three snacks per day.
5. Set aside a clothing allowance – you'll be needing new clothes!

3 Phase I: Reaching your target weight

Phase I is the dramatic stage of the Gi Diet when you will concentrate on losing the number of pounds you need to reach your target weight. During this period – whether it's 2 weeks or 2 months – you'll focus on eating green-light foods that are low-Gi and also low in fat and sugar. Yes, this means a farewell to cheesecake and a fond adieu to bacon. But it doesn't mean you can't have the occasional fling. Falling off the wagon, while not encouraged, is acceptable as long as it's the exception and not the rule. This diet is not a straitjacket. But if you do your best to eat the green-light way 90% of the time, you'll still lose weight. The odd lapse, at worst, will only delay you by a week or two from reaching your target weight.

There are six steps involved in getting launched on the green-light programme.

1. SET YOUR WEIGHT-LOSS TARGET

Before starting Phase I of your Gi Diet, there is one important preliminary step: setting your weight goals or targets. Since everyone has a distinct body type, metabolism and genes, there are no absolute rules for how much you should weigh. The only accepted international standard for weight is the **Body Mass Index (BMI)**, a measurement of how much body fat you are carrying relative to your height.

The BMI table on pages 32 to 33 is very simple to use. Just find your height in the chart in the horizontal column across the top and go down the table until you reach your weight. Where they intersect is your BMI, which is a pretty accurate estimate of the proportion of body fat you're carrying.

If your BMI falls between 19 and 24, your weight is within the acceptable norm. This is viewed as a healthy weight. Anything between 25 and 29 is considered overweight; and if you're 30 or over, you are officially obese.

Too thin or too heavy is not good. Your health is at risk if your BMI falls below 18.5 or above 25. As a woman, with a lower muscle mass and smaller frame than most men, you might want to target the lower end of the range, while men should generally target the higher end. However, if you are under 18 years, elderly or unusually muscle-bound – Serena Williams wouldn't fit on the chart! – these ratings do not apply to you. For those over 65, I suggest you allow an extra 10 pounds to help protect you in case of a fall, or as an extra energy reserve in case you get ill.

Of course, use this only as a guide, not as an absolute number. But it's a good ballpark figure, and the only one that has been accepted as an international standard.

The other measurement you should concern yourself with is your **waist measurement**. This is a even better predictor of your health than your weight. Abdominal fat is more than just a weight problem. Recent research has shown that abdominal fat acts almost like a separate organ in the body, except this 'organ' is a destructive one that releases harmful proteins and free fatty acids into the rest of the body, increasing your risk of life-threatening conditions, especially heart disease.

If you are female and have a waist measurement of 87.5cm (35in) or more, or male with a waist measurement of over 92.5cm (37in), you are at risk of endangering your health. Women with a measurement of 92.5cm (37in) or more or men with a measurement over 100cm (40in) are at serious risk of heart disease, stroke, many cancers and diabetes.

WEIGHT				HEIGHT																		
BRITISH		US		FT INS	4'6"	4'8"	4'10"	5'0"	5'2"	5'3"	5'4"	5'5"	5'6"	5'7"	5'8"	5'9"	5'10"	5'11"	6'0"	6'2"	6'4"	6'6"	6'8"
STONES	LBS	POUNDS	KILOS	CM	137	142	147	152	157	160	163	165	168	170	173	175	178	180	183	188	193	198	203
6	7	91	41		22.0	20.4	19.0	17.8	16.6	16.1	15.6	15.1	14.7	14.3	13.8	13.4	13.1	12.7	12.3	11.7	11.1	10.5	10.0
6	10	94	43		22.7	21.1	19.6	18.4	17.2	16.7	16.1	15.6	15.2	14.7	14.3	13.9	13.5	13.1	12.7	12.1	11.4	10.9	10.3
7	0	98	44		23.7	22.0	20.5	19.1	17.9	17.4	16.8	16.3	15.8	15.3	14.9	14.5	14.1	13.7	13.3	12.6	11.9	11.3	10.8
7	3	101	46		24.4	22.6	21.1	19.7	18.5	17.9	17.3	16.8	16.3	15.8	15.4	14.9	14.5	14.1	13.7	13.0	12.3	11.7	11.1
7	7	105	48		25.4	23.5	21.9	20.5	19.2	18.6	18.0	17.5	16.9	16.4	16.0	15.5	15.1	14.6	14.2	13.5	12.8	12.1	11.5
7	10	108	49		26.1	24.2	22.6	21.1	19.8	19.1	18.5	18.0	17.4	16.9	16.4	15.9	15.5	15.1	14.6	13.9	13.1	12.5	11.9
8	0	112	51		27.1	25.1	23.4	21.9	20.5	19.8	19.2	18.6	18.1	17.5	17.0	16.5	16.1	15.6	15.2	14.4	13.6	12.9	12.3
8	3	115	52		27.8	25.8	24.0	22.5	21.0	20.4	19.7	19.1	18.6	18.0	17.5	17.0	16.5	16.0	15.6	14.8	14.0	13.3	12.6
8	7	119	54		28.8	26.7	24.9	23.2	21.8	21.1	20.4	19.8	19.2	18.6	18.1	17.6	17.1	16.6	16.1	15.3	14.5	13.8	13.1
8	10	122	55		29.5	27.4	25.5	23.8	22.3	21.6	20.9	20.3	19.7	19.1	18.5	18.0	17.5	17.0	16.5	15.7	14.9	14.1	13.4
9	3	129	59		31.2	28.9	27.0	25.2	23.6	22.9	22.1	21.5	20.8	20.2	19.6	19.0	18.5	18.0	17.5	16.6	15.7	14.9	14.2
9	7	133	60		32.1	29.8	27.8	26.0	24.3	23.6	22.8	22.1	21.5	20.8	20.2	19.6	19.1	18.5	18.0	17.1	16.2	15.4	14.6
9	10	136	62		32.9	30.5	28.4	26.6	24.9	24.1	23.3	22.6	22.0	21.3	20.7	20.1	19.5	19.0	18.4	17.5	16.6	15.7	14.9
10	0	140	64		33.8	31.4	29.3	27.3	25.6	24.8	24.0	23.3	22.6	21.9	21.3	20.7	20.1	19.5	19.0	18.0	17.0	16.2	15.4
10	3	143	65		34.6	32.1	29.9	27.9	26.2	25.3	24.5	23.8	23.1	22.4	21.7	21.1	20.5	19.9	19.4	18.4	17.4	16.5	15.7
10	7	147	67		35.5	33.0	30.7	28.7	26.9	26.0	25.2	24.5	23.7	23.0	22.4	21.7	21.1	20.5	19.9	18.9	17.9	17.0	16.1
10	10	150	68		36.3	33.6	31.3	29.3	27.4	26.6	25.7	25.0	24.2	23.5	22.8	22.2	21.5	20.9	20.3	19.3	18.3	17.3	16.5
11	0	154	70		37.2	34.5	32.2	30.1	28.2	27.3	26.4	25.6	24.9	24.1	23.4	22.7	22.1	21.5	20.9	19.8	18.7	17.8	16.9
11	3	157	71		37.9	35.2	32.8	30.7	28.7	27.8	26.9	26.1	25.3	24.6	23.9	23.2	22.5	21.9	21.3	20.2	19.1	18.1	17.2
11	7	161	73		38.9	36.1	33.6	31.4	29.4	28.5	27.6	26.8	26.0	25.2	24.5	23.8	23.1	22.5	21.8	20.7	19.6	18.6	17.7
11	10	164	74		39.6	36.8	34.3	32.0	30.0	29.1	28.2	27.3	26.5	25.7	24.9	24.2	23.5	22.9	22.2	21.1	20.0	19.0	18.0
12	0	168	76		40.6	37.7	35.1	32.8	30.7	29.8	28.8	28.0	27.1	26.3	25.5	24.8	24.1	23.4	22.8	21.6	20.4	19.4	18.5
12	3	171	78		41.3	38.3	35.7	33.4	31.3	30.3	29.4	28.5	27.6	26.8	26.0	25.3	24.5	23.8	23.2	22.0	20.8	19.8	18.8
12	7	175	79		42.3	39.2	36.6	34.2	32.0	31.0	30.0	29.1	28.2	27.4	26.6	25.8	25.1	24.4	23.7	22.5	21.3	20.2	19.2

12	10	178	81		43.0	39.9	37.2	34.8	32.6	31.5	30.6	29.6	28.7	27.9	27.1	26.3	25.5	24.8	24.1	22.9	21.7	20.6	19.6
13	0	182	83		44.0	40.8	38.0	35.5	33.3	32.2	31.2	30.3	29.4	28.5	27.7	26.9	26.1	25.4	24.7	23.4	22.2	21.0	20.0
13	3	185	84		44.7	41.5	38.7	36.1	33.8	32.8	31.8	30.8	29.9	29.0	28.1	27.3	26.5	25.8	25.1	23.8	22.5	21.4	20.3
13	7	189	86		45.7	42.4	39.5	36.9	34.6	33.5	32.4	31.5	30.5	29.6	28.7	27.9	27.1	26.4	25.6	24.3	23.0	21.8	20.8
13	10	192	87		46.4	43.0	40.1	37.5	35.1	34.0	33.0	31.9	31.0	30.1	29.2	28.4	27.5	26.8	26.0	24.7	23.4	22.2	21.1
14	0	196	89		47.4	43.9	41.0	38.3	35.8	34.7	33.6	32.6	31.6	30.7	29.8	28.9	28.1	27.3	26.6	25.2	23.9	22.6	21.5
14	3	199	90		48.1	44.6	41.6	38.9	36.4	35.3	34.2	33.1	32.1	31.2	30.3	29.4	28.6	27.8	27.0	25.5	24.2	23.0	21.9
14	7	203	92		49.1	45.5	42.4	39.6	37.1	36.0	34.8	33.8	32.8	31.8	30.9	30.0	29.1	28.3	27.5	26.1	24.7	23.5	22.3
14	10	206	93		49.8	46.2	43.1	40.2	37.7	36.5	35.4	34.3	33.2	32.3	31.3	30.4	29.6	28.7	27.9	26.4	25.1	23.8	22.6
15	0	210	95		50.8	47.1	43.9	41.0	38.4	37.2	36.0	34.9	33.9	32.9	31.9	31.0	30.1	29.3	28.5	27.0	25.6	24.3	23.1
15	3	213	97		51.5	47.8	44.5	41.6	39.0	37.7	36.6	35.4	34.4	33.4	32.4	31.5	30.6	29.7	28.9	27.3	25.9	24.6	23.4
15	7	217	98		52.4	48.6	45.4	42.4	39.7	38.4	37.2	36.1	35.0	34.0	33.0	32.0	31.1	30.3	29.4	27.9	26.4	25.1	23.8
15	10	220	100		53.2	49.3	46.0	43.0	40.2	39.0	37.8	36.6	35.5	34.5	33.5	32.5	31.6	30.7	29.8	28.2	26.8	25.4	24.2
16	0	224	102		54.1	50.2	46.8	43.7	41.0	39.7	38.4	37.3	36.2	35.1	34.1	33.1	32.1	31.2	30.4	28.8	27.3	25.9	24.6
16	3	227	103		54.9	50.9	47.4	44.3	41.5	40.2	39.0	37.8	36.6	35.6	34.5	33.5	32.6	31.7	30.8	29.1	27.6	26.2	24.9
16	7	231	105		55.8	51.8	48.3	45.1	42.2	40.9	39.7	38.4	37.3	36.2	35.1	34.1	33.1	32.2	31.3	29.7	28.1	26.7	25.4
16	10	234	106		56.6	52.5	48.9	45.7	42.8	41.5	40.2	38.9	37.8	36.6	35.6	34.6	33.6	32.6	31.7	30.0	28.5	27.0	25.7
17	0	238	108		57.5	53.4	49.7	46.5	43.5	42.2	40.9	39.6	38.4	37.3	36.2	35.1	34.1	33.2	32.3	30.6	29.0	27.5	26.1
17	7	245	111		59.0	54.9	51.2	47.8	44.8	43.3	42.0	40.7	39.5	38.3	37.2	36.1	35.1	34.1	33.2	31.4	29.8	28.3	26.9
18	0	252	114		60.7	56.4	52.6	49.2	46.0	44.6	43.2	41.9	40.6	39.4	38.3	37.2	36.1	35.1	34.1	32.3	30.5	29.1	27.6
18	7	259	117		62.4	58.0	54.1	50.5	47.3	45.8	44.4	43.0	41.8	40.5	39.3	38.2	37.1	36.1	35.1	33.2	31.5	29.9	28.4
19	0	266	120		64.1	59.6	55.5	51.9	48.6	47.1	45.6	44.2	42.9	41.6	40.4	39.2	38.1	37.0	36.0	34.1	32.3	30.7	29.2
19	7	273	123		65.8	61.2	57.0	53.3	49.9	48.3	46.8	45.4	44.0	42.7	41.5	40.3	39.1	38.0	37.0	35.0	33.2	31.5	29.9
20	0	280	126		67.5	62.7	58.5	54.6	51.2	49.5	48.0	46.5	45.1	43.8	42.5	41.3	40.1	39.0	37.9	35.9	34.0	32.3	30.7

So I have your attention now! Make sure you measure correctly: put a tape measure around your waist at navel level till it fits snugly, without cutting into your flesh. Do not adopt the walking-down-the-beach-sucking-in-your-tummy stance. Just stand naturally. There's no point in trying to fudge the numbers, the only person you're kidding is yourself. Now you know your BMI and waist measurement you can set your weight target.

In Appendix V on page 254, we have inserted a Weight and Waist Log for you to keep track of the measurements you lose. This can be a powerful motivator, since nothing is more encourageing than success. Weigh and measure yourself weekly and do it at the same time of day, as even a bowel movement or a meal can add a pound or two at a time when every pound counts! An ideal time is first thing in the morning, before breakfast.

And don't get obsessed with numbers on the scale. Many people find themselves losing inches before they register any weight loss on the scales. Clothes start feeling a little looser, and before you know it you are down a dress size or getting into your old jeans. Soon you will probably have to buy new clothes. My readers often tell me that I should have warned them about the extra cost of refurbishing their wardrobe.

HOW LONG SHOULD IT TAKE?

Everyone who starts a diet is in a hurry to lose. And it's possible to drop weight – mostly water weight – quickly. But to keep the weight off, you must be patient.

If you are planning to lose up to 10% of your body weight (e.g. you weigh 10 stone and want to lose 1 stone), then you should plan on losing an average of 1lb per week. I say average because most people never lose weight in a straight line. The usual pattern is to lose more at the start of the diet, followed by a series of drops and plateaus. The closer you get to your target weight, the slower your weight loss will be. So for a 1 stone loss, assume this will take you 14 weeks.

If you have more than 10% to shed, the good news is that you will lose at a faster rate. This is simply because your larger body requires more calories just to keep operating than in the case of someone who is lighter.

Be prepared for slow, steady results. It took you a while to put on those extra pounds and it will take some time to lose them. Be patient and know that once that weight is gone, it will be gone forever as you keep it off in Phase II of the programme.

2. CLEAR OUT THE CUPBOARDS/PANTRY/FRIDGE

Take a look in your fridge. What do you see? Two jars of mayonnaise, some leftover Cheddar and a lot of sugar-laden condiments in jars? Now open the cupboards: what's the cookie and cracker situation? This is a good time to do an honest evaluation of what you tend to keep on hand. Consult the red-light columns and throw out anything that's on the list. Be ruthless. If you always have crisps on hand, let's face it – you will eat them. If you keep crackers around 'for the kids', you can be sure that they won't be the only ones snacking on them. If you hate waste, give the unopened food items and cans to your skinny neighbour or local food bank. When you banish red-light foods from your house, it will be a clear sign to your family that you're serious about eating the healthier, Gi way. (Getting your spouse and children on-board is discussed in detail in **Part II: The Family**.)

3. EAT BEFORE YOU SHOP

You know this one. Famished, you drop by the supermarket on your way home from work, and before you know it you've bought the biggest tray of cannelloni ever made. The worst mistake you can make is to go shopping on an empty stomach! You'll only be tempted to fill your cart with high-Gi, sugar-rich foods.

4. SHOP GREEN-LIGHT

Consult Chapter 4 to get some ideas of what you'd like to have for breakfast, lunch, dinner and snacks during your first week on the Gi Diet. Look through the recipe section at the end of the book and look at the Complete Gi Diet Food Guide on pages 234-47. (You could also pick up a copy of *The Gi Diet Guide to Shopping and Eating Out*.) Write out a shopping list and head to the supermarket. Your first few green-light shopping trips will require a bit more time and attention than usual as you familiarise yourself with green-light eating and meal planning. But don't worry, before long your new shopping and eating habits will become second nature.

Since it would be impossible to include every brand available in today's enormous supermarkets in the Gi Diet Food Guide, I've listed categories of food rather than individual brands, except in cases where clarification is needed, or there is an especially useful product available. This means that you will have to pay some attention to food labels. Some brands of the food I list in the green-light column may contain red-light ingredients, like sugar or trans fatty acids.

When reading a food label, there are six factors to consider when making the best green-light choice:

NUTRITION INFORMATION TYPICAL VALUES PER ½ PACKET
Energy 1237kJ/298kcal Protein 8.9g, Carbohydrate 17.5g, of which sugars 4.2g, Fat 21.3g, of which saturates 4.4g, Fibre 1.6g, Sodium 0.1g.
TYPICAL VALUES PER 100G
Energy 2474kJ/595kcal Protein 17.8g, Carbohydrate 35.0g, of which sugars 8.4g, Fat 42.6g, of which saturates 8.8g, Fibre 3.2g, Sodium 0.2g.

SERVING SIZE

Is the serving size realistic, or has the manufacturer lowered it so that the calories and fat levels will look better than the competition's? When comparing one brand with another, make sure you are comparing the same serving size.

CALORIES

Green-light means lower calories, so check this figure first. Sometimes products flagged as 'low-fat' still have plenty of calories, so don't be fooled by diet-friendly slogans on the front. Calories are calories, whether they come from fat or sugar.

FAT

Look at the amount of fat and the kind of fat. You want foods that are low-fat, with minimal or no saturated fats or trans fats. Remember that trans fats are often signalled by the phrases 'hydrogenated oils' or 'partially hydrogenated oils'.

FIBRE

Foods with lots of fibre have a low Gi, so this is an important component. When comparing brands, choose the one with higher fibre.

SUGAR

Most green-light foods are low in sugar. Again, watch for products that advertise themselves as 'low-fat', despite quietly bumping up the sugar content to make up for any perceived lost taste. Yogurts and cereals are good examples of this.

Sugars are sometimes listed as dextrose, glucose, fructose or sucrose – regardless of the form, it's sugar.

SODIUM

Sodium (salt) increases water retention, which doesn't help when you are trying to lose weight. It also contributes to premenstrual bloating in women and is a factor in hypertension (high blood pressure). Combine high blood pressure with excess weight and you move up to the front of the risk line for heart disease and stroke. So low-sodium products are preferable, because there is hidden salt in many processed products.

The Recommended Daily Allowance (RDA) for sodium in the UK is 1,500mg. The current average consumption is over 3,000 mg, so it goes without saying that most of us could stand to cut back on salt. However, if you have a BMI of over 30 and have any blood pressure, circulation or heart problems, you need to be even more vigilant about seeking out low-sodium brands. Canned products like soups are often high in sodium, as are many fast foods.

Dear Rick
My family doctor recommended your book The Gi Diet to me. After many years of trying many diets and diet groups I was never very successful. I may have lost a few pounds, but was not able to keep it off. On the Gi Diet, I have lost 1 1/2 stone and want to lose another 1 stone. I find the programme extremely easy to follow – it has become a way of life for me now. I like the way I feel – in control – and the way I look, and the confidence I now have. I'm determined to reach my target weight and show my friends and family the new me! My doctor says I'm his star patient.
Thank you, thank you!
Sincerely, Bobbi

5. EAT THE GREEN-LIGHT WAY

So you've restocked your pantry, and you've cracked the label codes. Now all you have to do on Phase I, the weight-loss phase, is stick to green-light foods and you're on your way. You will soon begin to feel better, your cravings will stop and it won't be long before you reach your target weight.

6. EXERCISE

Diet has far more impact on weight loss than exercise does. You can spend an hour on the treadmill and expend only 250 calories, which you can put right back on again if you eat half a large muffin on the way home. The following chart shows the amount of effort required to lose just one pound of fat.

EFFORT REQUIRED TO LOSE 1LB OF FAT

Exercise	9-stone person	11-stone person
Walking (4 mph – brisk)	53 miles/85km	42 miles/67km
Running (8-minute mile)	36 miles/58km	29 miles/46km
Cycling (12–14 mph)	96 miles/154km	79 miles/126km
Sex (average effort)	79 times	64 times

Not many of us are going to cycle 96 miles to go down a pound on the scales. But regular, moderate exercise is still very important in the long term, both for maintaining your new weight and for staying healthy. For example, if you were to walk briskly for half an hour a day 7 days a week, you would burn up calories equalling 9kg (20lb) of fat per year. This means that in Phase I, exercise is not essential to your weight-loss programme but it is an important consideration in Phase II, where you maintain your new weight. For women past the menopause, weight-bearing exercise is one way to counteract osteoporosis and the risk of fractures. And for families, exercising together – biking, skiing, whatever you enjoy – not only helps control weight but is also a way to enjoy each other's company.

Before you start shedding pounds, it might be hard to get out there and jog or hit the gym. But once you lose a bit of weight, being active will be something you crave and delight in. So stick with it – the fun will kick in eventually.

TYPES OF EXERCISE

Before we go any further, we should define exactly what we mean by exercise. There are three basic types of exercise, each working in a synergistic relationship with the others.

AEROBIC

The objective of aerobic exercise is to get your heart and lungs working harder. Aerobic exercise (walking, jogging, biking, swimming, hiking and so on) will have the most impact on your overall weight and health. In Chapter 11, there is more discussion about the impact of weight on your health, particularly heart disease, stroke and diabetes, which account for five deaths out of every ten.

STRENGTH

Strength training is particularly important as we move into middle age and beyond because of the steady reduction in muscle mass that accompanies ageing. Starting at the age of 25, the body loses 2% of its muscle mass each decade, a process that accelerates to 6–8% as we move into our senior years.

By exercising muscles on a regular basis, the loss can be minimised or reversed. And why is that important? Because the larger your muscles, the more energy (calories) they use. When you're at rest, or even asleep in bed, your muscles are using energy. So keeping or building muscle mass really helps you burn calories and lose weight.

Though regular exercise will help minimise muscle loss, it is through resistance exercises that we actually build muscle mass. Resistance exercises involve fixed or free weights, elastic bands or even your own body weight; pushing your hands together as hard as you can is a form of resistance exercise. You don't have to join a gym and work out with massive dumbbells. A few simple exercises, easily done at home, will do wonders to tone and restore those flabby muscles.

At the same time, strength training consumes calories. So whether at work or at rest, increased muscle mass helps you lose or maintain your weight.

STRETCHING

Again this is a significant issue as we age and lose flexibility in our joints, tendons and ligaments. Loss of flexibility reduces our ability to do either aerobic or strength training, both of which depend on healthy joints and tissues. In older people, this loss of flexibility can lead to falls and hip fractures. So although stretching may seem like a 'frill', it is central to the whole fitness picture.

Stretching exercises can give you noticeable results very quickly. Within just a week, you can increase your flexibility by over 100%. Both aerobic and strength training can actually make you less flexible if you don't stretch those muscle ligaments and tendons. That's why you always see athletes warming up and down with stretching exercises. So always include stretching, whether a simple set of muscle stretches or a yoga or t'ai chi session, in your exercise programme. (See page 47.)

Now let's review your options.

OUTDOOR ACTIVITIES

WALKING

This is by far the simplest and, for most people, the easiest exercise programme to start and maintain. For adults, 30 minutes a day 7 days a week should be your target. If you add 1 hour-long walk on the weekend, you can take a day off during the week. As mentioned before, we're talking about brisk walking, not speed walking nor ambling along. Imagine you're late for an appointment. The pace should increase your heart and breathing rates, but never to the point where you lack the breath to talk with a partner.

You don't need any special clothing or equipment, except a pair of comfortable cushioned shoes or sneakers. Walking is rarely boring since you can keep changing routes and watch the world go by. Walk with an older son or daughter for company and mutual support, or go solo and commune with nature and your own thoughts. If you have a child in a stroller, you can set a brisk pace that way, or invest in a jogger stroller. I prefer to walk on my own in the morning; this is when I do my best thinking of the day. This is not surprising when you realise how much extra oxygen-fresh blood is pumping through the brain.

A great idea for working people is to incorporate walking into the daily commute. I used to get off the bus three stops early on my way to and from work. Those three stops are equal to about 1 1/2 miles, so I was walking about 3 miles per day! If you drive to work, try parking your car about 1 1/2 miles away and walk to your job. You may even find cheaper parking farther away. However, start with just one stop early and work up. Who knows – distance permitting, you may eventually be able to walk to work. Think of the savings in petrol and parking fees!

JOGGING

This is similar to walking, but you need the proper footwear to protect joints from damage. The advantage of jogging over walking is that it approximately doubles the number of calories burned in the same period of time: 400 calories for jogging versus 200 for brisk walking over a 30-minute period. While walking, try jogging for a few yards and see if this is for you.

Jogging gets your heart rate up, which is great for heart health. The heart is basically a muscle and, like all muscles, it thrives on being exercised, so in general, the more the better. If jogging suits you, then this could be the simplest and most effective method of exercise as it uses personal time efficiently, can be done anytime, anywhere, and is inexpensive.

HIKING

Another variation on walking is cross-country hiking. Because this usually involves different kinds of terrain, especially hills and valleys, you use up more calories, about 50% more than for brisk walking. The reason for this is that you expend considerably more energy going uphill. Try hauling 65–90kg (140–200lb) up a hill and you'll get some idea of the extra effort your body has to make.

Hiking is fun, too, and is an especially good motivator for the whole family. It's an excuse for a special excursion out of town and for some adventure that can include every age, even a baby in a backpack. The only caveat is to choose a route that offers a variety of loops, from short to long. If your younger children flag, you can make your hikes suitable to the limits of the smallest. One way to satisfy everyone's level of fitness is to take turns: while you are with 'slow pack' – one parent plus the kids – your partner jogs or walks ahead, then loops back to join you and change over. This gives everyone a satisfying outing.

BICYCLING

Like walking, jogging and hiking, bicycling is a fun way to burn up calories, and it is almost as effective as jogging. For people with low-back or knee problems, it can be preferable. Other than the cost of the bike, it's inexpensive and can be done almost anywhere anytime, with helmets, plus lights, reflectors for night riding, of course.

SPORTS

Although most sports are terrific calorie burners, they usually cannot be part of a regular routine. Most of them require other people, equipment and facilities. But they can provide a boost to your regular fitness and exercise programme. Such popular sports as tennis, basketball, soccer, softball and golf (no golf cart, please) are excellent additions to a basic exercise programme. However, they're no substitute for a 5–7-day-a-week regular schedule.

INDOOR ACTIVITIES

Many of you will be muttering by now about how this would all be fine advice if we lived in Spain. But many of us must contend with either frigid, snowy winters or hot, humid summers, which limit outdoor activities.

The alternatives are either to organise a home gym or join a **fitness club**. The advantage of clubs is that they offer a wide range of sophisticated equipment, with instruction and advice from staff. Clubs are also social, and some people find they need group motivation to work out with enthusiasm. YMCAs also offer special programmes for the elderly, new mothers and those with special needs, and some provide subsidies for people who can't afford the membership fees. Many community centres offer free fitness classes, too.

If a fitness club isn't convenient or those Lycra-clad young things make you uncomfortable, you can always set up your exercise area at home. The best and least expensive piece of equipment is a **stationary bike**. The latest models work on magnetic resistance rather than the old friction strap around the flywheel. This gives a smoother action, with better tension adjustment. Most important, they are quiet, which is crucial if you want to be able to listen to music or watch TV. You can easily pay thousands for a bike with all the fancy trimmings, but the £125–£150 machines will work fine. Just be sure you choose one that has smooth, adjustable tension, then pop in that late-night movie or your favourite soap and get pedalling. You'll be amazed how quickly the minutes fly by: 20 minutes on the bike consumes the same number of calories as 30 minutes of brisk walking.

If biking is not for you, try a **treadmill**. These can be expensive, and beware of the lower-end models that cannot take the pounding. Expect to pay about £500 and up. Make sure the incline of the track can be raised and lowered for a better workout. Both treadmills and bikes can simulate outdoor walking, jogging, hiking or biking in the comfort of your own home. I use both of these machines but have added a **cross-country ski machine**, which has the advantage of working the upper body as well. Ski machines are generally less expensive than treadmills, but they cost more than stationary bikes. They also burn a higher number of calories (similar to jogging) because they use the arms and shoulders as well as the legs. It's almost the perfect all-body workout machine.

There are several other specialised options, such as stair climber machines, elliptical walkers and rowing machines, but they're not for everyone. They are also quite expensive, so make sure you try them out first at a fitness club or with a co-operative retailer.

STRENGTH TRAINING

It's now time to pay some attention to rebuilding your muscle mass. Remember that after the age of 40, you will lose between 1.8kg to 2.7kg (4–6lb) of muscle every decade, which is usually replaced with flab. That's 1.8kg to 2.7kg (4–6lb) of calorie-consuming muscle. Muscles burn up energy even when idle. Bigger muscles consume more energy than smaller muscles. So muscles come in handy for losing weight.

Resistance-training equipment can range from the complex and expensive to a £5 rubber band. Home gyms, with prices that begin at a couple of hundred pounds, are a popular option. For most people, however, there are cheaper, simpler methods, such as a set of free weights or (my own preference) rubber exercise bands such as Dyna-Band.

These resistance rubber bands and weights are available at many fitness exercise equipment retailers and surgical supply stores. Try a few resistance exercises, concentrating on the larger muscle groups – your legs, arms, and upper chest. These are the muscles that will give you the biggest bang by burning up the most calories. The resistance exercises should complement your other regular exercise regimen, not replace it. Committing to both types of exercise will produce far better results than either one alone. Resistance exercises are best done every other day, leaving time for your muscles to recuperate.

PILATES

I've recently become a pilates enthusiast. Originally, it was recommended by my physiotherapist to strengthen my back and prevent my disc problem from recurring. However, this very precise system of exercises does a lot more than just that. It's a series of floor exercises – no equipment needed – that both strengthen and stretch your muscles, especially the core muscles in your back and around your waist, which are essential for good posture. It's great for any level of fitness and at any age, and it is much less boring than step classes or other gym routines.

YOGA AND T'AI CHI

Yoga comes in different styles now: hatha, kundalini, kripalu, ashtanga, bikram and others. If you're new to yoga, the best choice is hatha, which teaches you simple postures that will keep you supple, offer relaxation techniques and improve your breathing and circulation. Ashtanga is trendy nowadays, but it is more aerobic and demanding. Kundalini focuses more on energising breathing techniques and meditation. But in any form, this ancient practice has much to offer, especially to anyone taking up exercise in middle age.

T'ai chi is another Eastern discipline that is gentle, promoting flexibility, balance and energy. It features a series of flowing postures, done standing, that many people like to practise early in the morning, out of doors. It keeps the joints and tendons supple, and offers a peaceful, revitalising form of activity that can carry you into old age. With both t'ai chi and yoga, there are a number of instructional DVDs or videos available for those who want to learn or practise at home.

As this is a book on nutrition, not exercise, I have not included any exercises for either stretching or strength training, particularly as there are a great number of excellent books on the subject. Check your local bookstore. Or you can consult the Web for free. For example, check out the BBC website at www.bbc.co.uk/health/healthy-living/fitness.

Follow these six steps and you will be on your way to your weight-loss goal. And don't despair if you fall off the wagon now and then. The mistake most people make is that one wrong move on a diet makes them feel so bad that they give up. You don't have to be that hard on yourself. If you're living on the programme 90% of the time, you will still successfully lose weight.

SUMMARY

The six steps to get you launched in Phase I are:
1. Set your weight/waist goal.
2. Clear the decks: pantry, fridge and freezer.
3. Eat before you shop.
4. Go green-light shopping and read your labels.
5. Eat the green-light way.
6. Include some exercise in your daily routine.

4 Meal basics

Let's break down what you can and can't eat for the three main meals and three snacks that are part of your daily Gi diet. Your alarm has rung, and now you're contemplating how to begin your day the green-light way. Let's start with breakfast.

BREAKFAST

I know you've been told that breakfast is the most important meal of the day. Well, it's true. It's the first thing you eat after your night-long 'fast' of 12 hours or more, and it launches you into your workday. The right sort of breakfast will help you avoid the need to grab a coffee and a Danish pastry as soon as you hit the office; it will send you off feeling light, energetic and well fed. And it doesn't mean you have to set the alarm any earlier either. If you have time to read the paper or feed the cat, you have time to prepare and eat a green-light breakfast.

The following chart lists all the typical breakfast foods according to the colour-coded categories. For a complete list of foods, see Appendix I on page 234. To ensure you have a balanced green-light breakfast, include some green-light carbohydrates, protein and fat.

Let's take a closer look at some of the usual breakfast choices.

COFFEE AND TEA

OK, this is the toughest one. The trouble with coffee is caffeine. It's not a health problem in itself, but it does stimulate the production of insulin. That's part of the 'buzz' we go looking for from coffee. But insulin reduces blood sugar levels, which then increases your appetite. Have you ever ordered a large coffee from Starbucks and then felt positively shaky an hour later? That's your blood sugar hitting bottom. You cure it by eating – which is when a muffin seems like the only choice.

This caffeine cycle is not helpful when you're trying to keep your appetite stable and under control. So in Phase I, try to cut out coffee altogether. As unpleasant as it is, caffeine withdrawal is over in a day or two. First, cut down on quantity, from medium to small; then try a half-caffeinated, half-decaf blend. Or you can limit yourself to decaffeinated coffee – some taste as good as the real thing. Even better, switch to tea. It has only about a third of the caffeine of coffee, and black tea has health benefits as well: it's rich in antioxidants, and beneficial for heart health and reducing the risk of dementias. Green tea is also considered an anti-carcinogen. (My 95-year-old mother and her tea-drinking cronies are living proof!) Herbal teas, such as peppermint, chamomile and other blends, are fine too, as long as they contain no caffeine. But if coffee is going to be a deal breaker, then go ahead, have one cup a day, but not a double espresso. If you take milk and sugar, make it skimmed milk and a sweetener such as Splenda®.

CEREALS

Another toughie. Most cold cereals contain hidden or not-so-hidden sugars, and are red-light. The green-light ones are high in fibre – at least 10g per serving. All right, they're not a lot of fun by themselves, but you can liven them up with fresh, canned or frozen fruits, a few nuts or some fruit yogurt (fat-free, with sweetener).

My personal favourite is good old-fashioned oatmeal – not

the instant type in packets but the large-flake, slow-cooking kind. (They're starting to serve it in the smartest hotels now.) It really does 'stick to your ribs', as my mother used to say. Not only is large-flake oatmeal low-Gi, but it's also low-calorie and has been shown to lower cholesterol. Yes, you have to cook it, but this takes about 3 minutes or so in the microwave. Dress it up with yogurt, sliced almonds, berries or unsweetened applesauce. It's also just fine with nothing but milk on it. I probably receive more emails about people's delight in rediscovering oatmeal than about any other food or meal. Give it a try.

TOAST

Go ahead, but no more than one slice a meal. Make sure you choose bread that has at least 2.5–3g of fibre per slice. (Note: Most breads quote a two-slice serving, which should equal 5–6g per serving.) The best choice is 100% stone-ground wholemeal bread. This has a coarser grind, and therefore a lower Gi. White bread, cracked wheat or anything else made with white flour is red-light.

BUTTER AND JAMS

Butter is out. It's very high in saturated fat, and despite the protestations of the dairy industries, it's not good for your health or waistline. Yes, it does make things taste good – that's what fat does best! But you can still enjoy any one of a variety of light non-hydrogenated soft margarines, if you use only a teaspoon or so.

For jams, look for the 'extra fruit/no sugar added' varieties. Fruit, not sugar, should be the first ingredient listed. They taste great and don't have the calories of the usual commercial jams.

BREAKFAST For complete food listings see appendix 1, p. 234

	RED	YELLOW	GREEN
PROTEIN			
Meat and Eggs	Regular bacon Sausages	Turkey bacon Omega-3 eggs (Columbus)	Back bacon, Lean ham Egg whites
Dairy	Milk (whole) Cheese Yoghurt (full-fat) Cottage cheese (full-fat) Cream Goats milk	Milk (semi-skimmed) Cream cheese (light) Yoghurt (low-fat with sugar)	Milk (skimmed) Cheese (fat-free) Fruit yoghurt (fat-free with sweetener e.g. Muller Lite) Cottage cheese (low-fat or fat-free) Buttermilk, low-fat Soya milk, plain, low-fat

CARBOHYDRATES

Cereals	All cold cereals except those listed as yellow- or green-light Muesli (branded)	Shredded Wheat Bran	Porridge (large-flake 'old-fashioned' oats) Alpen Crunchy Bran All-Bran Fibre 1 Home-made Muesli High-Fibre Bran Oat bran 100% Bran
Breads/ Grains	White bread Bagels Baguette Croissants Doughnuts Muffins Pancakes/Waffles Biscuits Crispbreads (regular) Melba toast	Whole grain breads*	100% stone-ground wholemeal (Warburtons)* Wholegrain, high-fibre breads (2½–3g. fibre/slice) Crispbreads, high-fibre*

Limited portions. See p.25

	RED	YELLOW	GREEN
Fruits	All dried fruit All canned fruits in syrup Canteloupe Melons Watermelon	Raisins Bananas Fruit cocktail in juice Apricots (fresh and dried) Pineapple	Apples Peaches Pears Oranges Grapefruit Plums Grapes Berries (all)
Juices	Prune All sweetened juices All fruit drinks	Apple (unsweetened) Grapefruit (unsweetened) Orange (unsweetened) Pear (unsweetened)	Eat the fruit, rather than drink its juice
Vegetables*	French fries Hash browns		Most vegetables*

*See p. 234 for complete list.

FATS

Butter Hard margarine Peanut butter (regular and light) Tropical oils Vegetable fat	Soft margarine (non-hydrogenated) Vegetable oil 100 % Peanut butter**	Soft margarine (non-hydrogenated light)** Rapeseed oil** Olive oil** Almonds** Hazelnuts** Vegetable oil sprays

***Limited portions. See p.25*

DAIRY FOODS

Low-fat dairy products are an ideal green-light choice and an excellent source of protein. I have a glass of skimmed milk every morning. I admit that skimmed didn't taste great at first, but I weaned myself by switching to 1% before moving to skimmed. Now 2% tastes like cream!

Fat-free yogurt with sweetener instead of sugar is ideal for breakfast, dessert or a snack, either by itself or added to fruits or cereals.

Low-fat cottage cheese is also a top-rated green-light source of protein. Or you can make a low-fat soft cheese spread by letting yogurt drain in cheesecloth overnight in the refrigerator.

Regular, full-fat dairy products, including whole milk and cream, cheese and butter are loaded with saturated fat and should be avoided completely.

EGGS

Whole eggs are a yellow-light food. The best option is omega-3 eggs (e.g. Columbus) as omega-3 is good for a healthy heart. Otherwise, use egg whites. If you're eating a hotel breakfast, in most cases the kitchen is happy to make omelettes with egg whites only.

BACON

Bacon is red-light because of its high saturated fat content. However, there are tasty green-light alternatives, such as back bacon, turkey bacon and lean ham.

LUNCH

Lunch is usually the most problematic meal because we're at the mercy of other factors – we tend to eat this meal outside the home and in a hurry. So lunch takes a little strategising. You have two options: make a packed lunch, packing items from your green-light pantry, or eat at a restaurant, take away or fast-food outlet.

THE LUNCH BOX OPTION

Bringing your own lunch to work is the easiest way to eat green-light. And if you're a mother or father who already has to pack school lunches, all you have to do is assemble one more, for you. And there are other advantages to lunching in, besides avoiding the temptation of a red-light lunch: it's cheaper, and it gives you downtime at your desk to read or catch up on paperwork.

SANDWICHES

Sandwiches are the lunchtime staple, and it's no wonder: they're portable, easy to make and offer endless variety. They can also be a dietary disaster, but if you follow the suggestions below you can keep your sandwiches green-light.

- Always use 100% stone-ground wholemeal or high-fibre whole grain bread (2½–3g fibre per slice).
- Sandwiches should be served open-faced. Either pack components separately and assemble just before eating or make your sandwich with a 'lettuce lining' that helps keep the bread from getting soggy. Then discard the extra slice (or share it with the birds).
- Include at least three vegetables, such as lettuce, tomato, red or green pepper, cucumber, sprouts or onion.

LUNCH: For complete food listings see appendix 1, p. 234

	RED	YELLOW	GREEN
PROTEIN			
Meat and Eggs	Hot dogs Hamburgers Minced beef (regular) Sausages Processed meats	Lamb (lean cuts) Pork (lean cuts) Ground beef (lean) Omega-3 eggs (Columbus) Milk (semi-skimmed) Cheese (low-fat) Yoghurt (low-fat with sugar) Cream cheese (light) Crème fraiche (low-fat)	All fish and seafood, fresh or frozen (no batter or breading) or canned (in water) Pork tenderloin Beef (Top/Eye round beef steak) Lean deli ham Quorn Chicken breast (skinless) Turkey breast (skinless) Veal Minced beef (extra lean) Egg whites
Dairy	Milk (whole) Cheese Yoghurt (full-fat) Cottage cheese (full-fat) Cream cheese Chocolate milk		Milk (skimmed) Cottage cheese (low-fat or fat-free) Fruit yoghurt (fat-free with sweetener) Ice cream (low-fat with no sugar added) Sour cream (fat-free)

CARBOHYDRATES

Breads/ Grains	White bread Baguette/Croissants Crispbreads Rice cakes Croutons Couscous Rice (short grain, white, easy-cook) Pancakes/ Waffles Cake/Biscuits Muffins/Doughnuts Macaroni cheese Gnocchi Noodles Ravioli with cheese Tortellini with cheese Pizza Hamburger buns	Wholegrain breads* Pitta (Wholemeal) Crispbread with fibre	100% stone-ground wholemeal* Wholegrain, high-fibre breads* (2.5g–3g fibre/slice) Crispbreads high-fibre* Pasta* (fettuccine, spaghetti, penne, vermicelli, linguine, macaroni) Rice (basmati, wild, brown, long-grain)

*Limit portions. See p. 25

	RED	YELLOW	GREEN
FRUIT	Melons All dried fruit Cantaloupe	Bananas Apricots Kiwi Pineapple Papaya	Apples Oranges Pears Grapefruit Peaches Plums Grapes Strawberries Blueberries Raspberries Blackberries Rhubarb Avocado (1/4)
VEGETABLES **Limit portions, see p. 25*	Potatoes (mashed or baked) French fries Parsnips Swede Turnips	Potatoes (boiled) Corn Squash Sweet potatoes Beetroot Artichoke	Potatoes (boiled new)* Asparagus Broccoli Cauliflower Peas Courgettes Aubergine Mushrooms Mangetout Celery Onions Spinach Cabbage Lettuce Tomatoes Cucumbers Peppers Olives* Pickles
BEANS/LEGUMES **see p.234 for complete list*	Baked beans with pork Broad beans Refried beans		Most beans

FATS	Butter Peanut Butter (regular and light) Hard margarine Tropical oils Vegetable fat Cheese Mayonnaise Salad dressings (regular)	Soft margarine (non-hydrogenated) 100% Peanut butter* Most nuts* Mayonnaise (light) Salad dressings (light)	Soft margarine (non-hydrogenated, light)* Rapeseed oil* Olive oil* Almonds* Mayonnaise (fat-free) Salad dressings (fat-free, low-sugar) Vinaigrette
SOUPS	All cream-based soups Tinned split pea Tinned green pea Tinned black bean Puréed vegetable	Tinned Lentil Tinned Tomato Tinned Chicken noodle	Chunky bean, vegetable and pasta soups (e.g. Baxter's Healthy Choice) All home-made soups made with green-light ingredients

*Limited portions. See p.25

- Instead of spreading with butter or margarine, use mustard or hummus.
- Add up to 100g (4oz) of cooked lean meat or fish – roast beef, turkey, shrimp or salmon.
- For tuna or chicken salad, use low-fat mayonnaise or low-fat salad dressing and celery.
- Mix tinned salmon with malt vinegar or fresh lemon.

SALADS

Preparing salads may seem more labour-intensive than sandwiches, but it doesn't have to be. Invest in a variety of plastic containers so you can pack them easily. Keep a supply of green-light vinaigrette on hand, wash greens ahead of time and store in paper towels in plastic bags. You'll find that creative salads are a good way to use up leftovers with a minimum of fuss.

Basic salad

Makes 1 serving

90g (3oz) lettuce, such as cos, leaf, butterhead or iceberg lettuce, mesclun, rocket, watercress or baby spinach, torn or coarsely chopped
1 small carrot, grated
1/2 red, yellow or green pepper, diced
1 plum tomato, cut into wedges
75g (2 1/2oz) sliced cucumber
40g (1 1/2oz) chopped red onion (optional)

1. In a bowl, toss together the lettuce, carrot, pepper, tomato, cucumber and onion.
2. Dress your salad with about 1 tbsp Basic Vinaigrette (recipe

below). Be vigilant with salad dressing: use either 1tbsp of the recipe below or the same amount of a low-fat, low-sugar, store-bought dressing.

VARIATIONS: You can make a meal out of this salad by adding 100g (4oz) canned tuna, cooked salmon, tofu, kidney beans, chickpeas, cooked chicken or another lean meat.
STORAGE: A good way to keep greens fresh is to wash them when you buy them, dry thoroughly and wrap loosely in paper towels (newspapers actually work well, too), then store in the crisper. Having washed greens on hand makes daily salad preparation easier.

Basic Green-light Vinaigrette

2 tbsp vinegar, such as white or red wine vinegar, balsamic, rice or cider (or you can use lemon juice)
1 tbsp extra-virgin olive oil or rapeseed oil
1/2 tsp Dijon mustard
Pinch salt
Pinch freshly ground black pepper
Pinch dried or fresh herbs (thyme, oregano, basil, marjoram, mint or Italian seasoning)
1 clove garlic, crushed (optional)

1. In a small bowl, whisk together the vinegar, oil, mustard, salt, pepper, herbs and garlic, or shake it all together in a small glass jar with tight-fitting lid.

STORAGE: Both the salad and the dressing can be prepared ahead and stored, separately, covered, for about 2 days.

Salade Niçoise

Makes 1 serving

2 small new potatoes, skins on, cooked and quartered
120g (4oz) green beans, briefly cooked
60g (2oz) torn or coarsely chopped lettuce
1 tbsp green-light vinaigrette or other low-fat dressing
55g (2oz) tinned tuna, drained and flaked
1 hard-boiled egg, peeled and quartered
1 medium tomato, quartered
1 anchovy fillet (optional)
6 pitted black olives
Chopped fresh parsley
Salt and freshly ground black pepper

1. In a serving bowl, combine the potatoes, beans and lettuce. Add vinaigrette and toss gently.
2. Place tuna in centre and arrange wedges of egg and tomato around it.
3. Add the anchovy, if using, and the olives.
4. Sprinkle with parsley.
5. Season with salt and pepper to taste.

FRESH TUNA OPTION: Substitute grilled fresh tuna for the tinned tuna.

Waldorf Chicken and Rice Salad

Makes 1 serving

50g (1 3/4oz) basmati or brown rice
1 medium apple, chopped

1 or 2 stalks celery, chopped
30g (1oz) walnuts, chopped
100 g (4 oz) cooked chicken (page 73), chopped
1 tbsp store-bought light buttermilk dressing, or dressing made with half low-fat yogurt, half low-fat mayonnaise

1. Cook the rice, drain and leave to cool.
2. In a bowl, combine the cooked rice, apple, celery, walnuts and chicken. Mix in the dressing. Keep refrigerated until serving.

Basic Pasta Salad Lunch

Makes 1 serving

40g (1 1/2oz) wholemeal pasta (spirals, shells or similar shape)
125g (5oz) chopped cooked vegetables (broccoli, asparagus, peppers, courgette, spring onions – whatever's on hand)
60ml (2fl oz) light tomato sauce or any low-fat/non-fat pasta sauce
100g (4oz) chopped cooked chicken, ground turkey or lean chicken sausage

1. Cook the pasta, drain and leave to cool.
2. In a large bowl, combine the cooked pasta, vegetables, sauce and chicken. Keep refrigerated until serving. Serve either warmed in the microwave or chilled.

VEGETARIAN OPTION: Use soy-based ground meat substitute instead of the chicken or turkey.

Cottage Cheese and Fruit

Makes 1 serving

225g (8oz) low-fat cottage cheese
100g (4oz) diced fresh fruit or fruit canned in juice only (peaches, apricots or pears)
Sliced almonds or a few pecans (optional)

1. In a plastic container, combine the cottage cheese, fruit and nuts, if using. Seal with a tight-fitting lid.

VARIATION: Add 1tbsp double-fruit, no-added-sugar jam instead of the chopped fruit.

LET'S GO OUT FOR LUNCH

Having lunch at a restaurant is tricky. Your friends may tempt you with their orders of fries and pizza. Bringing your own lunch is definitely the best option – and easier on the budget, too. But you don't want to sit at your desk with a brown bag every day, so here are some strategies for running the dining-out gauntlet.

EATING THE GI WAY IN RESTAURANTS

Here are nine tips for keeping your restaurant luncheon meal low-Gi:

- Drink a glass of water before you order or eat. It helps prevent overeating.
- Ignore the breadbasket. Flatbreads may look thin and diet-ish but, like crackers, they often have hidden trans fats, and they are not low-calorie. Bread rolls are white flour incarnate. Take a pass.

- A good addition to your main course is a chunky bean or vegetable-based soup. But avoid cream-based, noodle or puréed-vegetable soups.
- As it is virtually impossible to get new/small boiled potatoes, always ask for double vegetables in lieu. I've requested this hundreds of times and have never been refused.
- If you order rice, look for long-grain, brown or wild rice. Avoid sticky white rice. The portion should only cover one quarter of your plate.
- The only problem with ordering pasta is the size of the portions most restaurants serve. It shouldn't form the base of the meal. Eat the Italian way, treating pasta as a modest first course or a side dish. Italians are appalled at the vast bowls of pasta we consume. Order wholemeal pasta, if available. Most restaurants aren't geared to serving smaller portions, but ask for a half portion or order one portion and split it with friend.
- Avoid sauces, except for low-fat ones such as tomato and basil. No creamy alfredo!
- When ordering a salad, ask them to serve the dressing on the side, then use only a spoonful of it. Avoid coleslaws, potato salads or anything made with mayonnaise.
- If there's a choice between sautéed and grilled, always go for grilled. Sautéeing usually involves oils or butter. And skip the breaded schnitzels and the tempura shrimp.
- Eat slowly. Put your fork down between bites. It takes up to half an hour for your stomach to tell your brain when it's had enough. Rushing meals is the most common cause of overeating.
- Best to skip dessert and enjoy a green-light yogurt when you're back at work. Most conventional desserts are red light and even 'diet' desserts will deliver calories.

FAST FOOD

A couple of years ago, the idea of getting a green-light meal at a fast-food restaurant was simply laughable. Now, partly due to the threat of legal action and a stagnant market share, the major fast-food chains are finally offering some healthy options. Subway, for instance, has pioneered the move to healthy choices for some time, and it has been reflected in their successful growth.

Although things are changing in McDonald's land, fast food is still a minefield. Pizza is red-light all the way thanks to its high-Gi crust and the saturated fat in the cheese toppings. Beef burgers are also soaked in saturated fat as are breaded, deep-fried chicken and fish. And all the trimmings – fries, ketchup, milkshakes and fizzy drinks – are loaded with fat and sugar. Still, there are a few points of light in this sea of gloom, and I've listed them below. I have put an asterisk beside items that are excessively high in sodium – the fast food industry frequently boosts salt content when they lower the fat in their products to make up for any perceived loss of flavour which, as we know, can be hazardous to your health.

Ground rules

1. Always eat burgers open-faced and throw away the top half of the bun.
2. Always ask for low-fat dressings and use half of the sachet.

McDonald's

Salads

- Grilled Chicken Caesar Salad (hold the croutons)
- Grilled Chicken Ranch Salad

Sandwiches/Burgers

- Low-fat Grilled Chicken
- Grilled Chicken Flat Bread
- Quorn Premiere

Snacks

- Oatso Simple & Jam
- Fruit and Yogurt

Burger King

Salads

- Flame Grilled Chicken Salad
- Warm Crispy Chicken Salad
- Premium Caesar Salad

Burgers/Sandwiches

- Piri Piri Chicken Baguette*
- Flame Grilled Chicken Sandwich

Snacks

- Twin Pot Bio Yogurt
- Twin Pot Fresh Fruit

Dressings

- Honey and Mustard
- Tomato and Basil
- French

Subway

Sandwiches (6in under 6g fat subs)

- Ham*
- Honey Mustard Ham*
- Roast Beef*
- Roast Chicken Breast

- Subway Club*
- Sweet Onion and Chicken Teriyaki*
- Turkey Breast*
- Turkey Breast, Ham and Roast Beef*
- Veggie Delite

Deli Subs

- Ham Deli
- Roast Beef Deli
- Turkey Breast Deli

Salads

- Garden Fresh (Side Salad)
- Mediterranean Chicken

Dressings

- Fat-free Honey Mustard
- Fat-free Sweet Onion

Wraps

- Grilled Chicken
- Turkey Breast

Prêt a Manger

Sandwiches

- Slim Prêt – Hummus and Tomato
- Slim Prêt – Crayfish and Rocket
- Fresh Herb Chicken No Mayo
- No Bread Tuna Sandwich

Salads

- Ham Salad Mayo Frais
- Chicken Salad Mayo Frais
- No Bread Chicken Caesar

Other Fast Food Chains

If you go into other fast food outlets, such as Tesco Express, Sainsbury Local, Marks & Spencer, Benjys etc. steer clear of sandwiches and rolls containing mayonnaise and cheese. Look for wholemeal and high-fibre breads and eat them open faced.

Sandwich bars

Sandwich bars are an excellent alternative to fast-food outlets as they enable you to customise your sandwich and see exactly what is going into it. Here is what to ask for to ensure your sandwich is green light:

- Wholemeal or granary bread
- Hummus or mustard in lieu of butter, margarine or mayonnaise
- Lean slices of chicken or turkey breast, ham or tuna as the principal filling. Avoid mayonnaise, cheese and bacon bits
- Add lots of vegetables such as tomatoes, avocado, lettuce, salad leaves or onion rings for flavour and nutrition
- Always remove the top slice of bread and eat the sandwich open faced.

This information was correct at time of going to press. However, as this is a dynamic field, you may wish to check these restaurants' menus or websites from time to time to see if they have expanded their green-light offerings. Every restaurant usually has nutritional breakdowns available for its menu items, if you ask for them.

DINNER

At the end of the day, we may have more time to eat – and to overeat. And the fatigue that arrives towards the end of the day is an encouragement to eat too much. There's also a tradition of eating more at dinner, despite the fact that most people will simply go to bed on a full stomach rather than be active in the evening. Family dinners can present challenges, too: sometimes the designated cook has to feed two shifts – children first, then late-arriving partners. This means more time in the kitchen and more time waiting, making it tempting to graze and snack.
So with the pitfalls of dinner in mind, here is our traffic chart listing popular dinnertime foods. Remember that you can find a full list of foods in Appendix I, page 234.

PROTEIN

This part of your dinner should cover no more than one-quarter of your plate (assuming you don't use huge plates!). A serving size should be 100g (4oz) – it should cover no more than the palm of your hand and be roughly the thickness of your hand.

Red meat

This is allowed, but most red meat contains saturated fat. However, there are a few ways to minimise the fat.

- Buy only low-fat meats such as top round beef. For hamburgers or spaghetti sauces, buy extra-lean minced beef. Veal or pork tenderloin are low-fat, too. As for juicy steaks, well, they are juicy because of the fat in them, so they're not a good choice.
- Trim any visible fat. Just 5mm (1/4in) of fat can double the total amount of fat in the meat.

- Broiling or grilling allows the excess fat from the meat to drain off. (Try a George Foreman-style fat-draining electric grill.)
- For cooking on the hob, use a non-stick pan, with a vegetable oil spray, rather than try to fry with a teaspoon of oil. The spray goes further.

Poultry

Chicken and turkey breast – *without the skin* – are excellent green-light choices. In the yellow-light category are skinless thighs, wings and legs, which are higher in fat.

Seafood

Always a good green-light choice. Although certain cold-water fish such as salmon and cod have a relatively high oil content, fish oil is beneficial to your heart health. Shrimp and squid are fine, too, as long as they aren't breaded or battered. Fish and chips, alas, are out.

Beans (legumes)

If you're not a 'bean person', it's time to re-evaluate! Beans are such a good source of so many good Gi things: fibre, low-fat protein, and complex carbs that deliver nutrients while taking their time going through the digestive system. And they are a snap to incorporate into salads and soups to add your quotient of protein. Chickpeas, lentils, white (flageolet) beans, black beans, kidney beans – a bean for every day of the week. But watch out for canned pork and beans; it's high in sugar and fat. And avoid canned bean soups, where the processing has increased the overall Gi rating.

You will find several delicious recipes using beans in the Recipes section.

DINNER: For complete food listings see appendix 1, p. 234

	RED	YELLOW	GREEN
PROTEIN			
Meat and Eggs	Minced beef (regular) Hamburgers Hot dogs Sausages Processed meats	Minced beef (lean) Lamb (Fore/Legshank, centre cut, loin chop) Boiled ham Pork (tenderloin, loin chop) Chicken/turkey leg (skinless) Beef (sirloin steak, sirloin tip) Omega 3 eggs (Columbus)	Pork tenderloin Minced beef (extra lean) Fish (without batter) Shellfish Lean deli ham Chicken breast (skinless) Turkey breast (skinless) Veal Beef (top round/eye round) Egg whites (Columbus)
Dairy	Cheese Milk (whole) Chocolate milk Yoghurt (full-fat) Cottage cheese (full-fat) Sour cream (full-fat) Ice-cream	Cheese (low-fat) Crème fraiche (low-fat) Yoghurt (low-fat with sugar) Frozen yoghurt (low-fat, low-sugar) Ice-cream (low-fat) Milk (semi-skimmed)	Fruit yoghurt (fat-free with sweetener) Cottage cheese (low-fat or fat-free) Back-bacon Buttermilk (low-fat) Ice-cream (low-fat, no sugar added) Milk (skimmed) Soy milk plain, low-fat

CARBOHYDRATES			
Breads/ Grains	White bread Crispbreads Baguette/ Croissants Bagels Cake/Biscuits Doughnuts/Muffins Pancakes/Waffles Gnocchi Macaroni cheese Rice (easy-cook) Pizza Tortillas Noodles Tortellini with cheese or meat Cereal/granola bars Tortillas Melba toast	Wholegrain breads Pitta (wholemeal) Crispbread with fibre	100% stone-ground wholemeal* Rice* (basmati, wild, brown, long-grain) Pasta* (fettuccine, spaghetti, penne, vermicelli, linguine, macaroni) Pumpernickel bread* Wholegrain high-fibre (2.5–3g fibre/slice Crispbreads, high fibre
**Limit portions. See p. 25*			
PASTA SAUCES	Pasta sauces Alfredo Sauces with added meat or cheese Sauces with added sugar or sucrose	Sauces with vegetables	Light sauces with or without vegetables (no added sugar)

	RED	YELLOW	GREEN	
FRUIT	Raisins Dates Watermelon Cantaloupe	Bananas Apricots (fresh dried) Kiwi Pineapple Papaya Mangoes Cranberries (dried)	Apples Oranges Pears Grapefruit Peaches Plums Grapes Cherries Strawberries	Blueberries Raspberries Blackberries Rhubarb Cranberries Apple sauce (sugar-free e.g. Clearspring Organic) Apple purée
VEGETABLES ** Limited portions see p.25*	Potatoes(mashed or baked) French fries	Potatoes(boiled) Corn	Potatoes (boiled, new)* Asparagus Broccoli Cauliflower Beans (green/ runner) Peas Courgette Aubergine Mushrooms	Mangetout Celery Onions Spinach Cabbage Lettuce Tomatoes Cucumbers Peppers Pickles Olives*
BEANS/LEGUMES	Broad beans		Black Black-eyed Butter Chickpeas	Lima Mung Pigeon Pinto

			Haricot/Navy Italian Kidney Lentils Romano Soy Split
TINNED BEANS	Baked beans w. pork Refried beans		Baked beans (low-fat) Mixed salad beans Vegetarian chilli
FATS	Butter Lard Vegetable fat Hard margarine Tropical oils Peanut butter (all varieties) Mayonnaise Salad dressings (regular)	Soft margarine (non-hydrogenated) Hazelnuts* Mayonnaise (light) Salad dressings (light) Most vegetable oils* Most nuts*	Soft margarine, (non-hydrogenated, light)* Rapeseed oil* Olive oil* Mayonnaise (fat-free) Salad dressings (low-fat/sugar) Vinaigrette, (low-sugar) Vegetable oil sprays Almonds

*Limit portions See p.25

	RED	YELLOW	GREEN
SOUPS	All cream-based soups Tinned split pea Tinned green pea Tinned black bean Tinned puréed vegetable	Tinned lentil Tinned tomato Tinned chicken noodle	Chunky bean, vegetable and pasta (e.g. Baxter's Healthy Choice) All home-made soups using green-light ingredients (see recipes p.230)
BEVERAGES **In phase II a glass of wine and the occasional beer may be included*	Alcoholic drinks* Fruit drinks Milk (whole) Regular coffee Regular soft drinks Sweetened juice	Diet soft drinks (caffeinated) Milk (semi-skimmed) Red wine* Regular coffee (with skimmed milk, no sugar) Unsweetened fruit juices: Apple Cranberry Grapefruit Orange Pear Pineappple	Bottled water Tonic water Decaffeinated coffee (with skimmed milk, no sugar) Diet soft drinks (no caffeine) Herbal teas Light instant chocolate Milk (skimmed) Tea (with skimmed milk, no sugar)

Soy (tofu)

You don't have to be vegetarian to enjoy soy, which is low in saturated fat and an excellent source of protein. While tofu is not a thriller on its own, it 'cooks up well', and takes on the flavours of whatever dishes it is added to. Seasoned tofu scrambles, for instance, are a good substitute for scrambled eggs. Choose soft tofu, which has up to a third less fat than the firm variety.

Textured vegetable protein (TVP)

This is not a new device for prerecording TV shows! TVP is a soy alternative to meat that looks a lot like minced beef, and can be used in the same ways – in lasagne, chilli, stir-fry and spaghetti sauce. It's quite tasty and delivers the texture of meat. Our middle son, a vegetarian who has since left the nest, put us onto this adaptable product.

POTATOES, PASTA, RICE

These are the ones that veteran dieters have been conditioned to avoid. But they are fine as long as they only cover one-quarter of the plate.

Remember, with potatoes your first choice is boiled small, preferably new, potatoes. All other choices, especially baked potatoes or French fries, are red-light. Incidentally, although sweet potatoes are not technically potatoes, they are a good lower-Gi food. But since they tend to come in larger sizes, I suggest you save these for Phase II.

If you want to make sure that you get the pasta portion right, measure 40g (1 1/2oz) uncooked pasta. And remember to undercook it a little so that it is slightly firm to the bite (*al dente*). For rice, stick to 50g (1 3/4oz) uncooked basmati, wild, brown or long-grain rice.

VEGETABLES

Here you can put the scales away. Eat as many vegetables and as much salad as you like; they should be the backbone of your meal. Always include at least two vegetables. Experiment with something you've never had before. Baby pak choi is delicious grilled, and rapini, a dark green vegetable that looks like broccoli with more leaves, is a nice change. The dark, curly green vegetables such as kale have a strong taste and are full of good things, including folic acid.

Greens such as rocket or baby spinach come conveniently prewashed in bags. Frozen bags of mixed vegetables are inexpensive and convenient; you can even toss the veggies into a saucepan, add tomato juice with a dollop of salsa and you have a quick vegetable soup.

DESSERTS

Yes, desserts are indeed part of the Gi Diet – at least, the ones that are green-light and good for you. This includes most fruits, and low-fat, low-sugar dairy products, such as fruit yogurt and ice cream. The recipe section (page 182) offers several truly satisfying desserts, such as Apple Raspberry Coffee Cake, or Frozen Ricotta Treat.

DINING OUT

Dining out on the Gi Diet is not difficult since many restaurants have made the switch to olive or vegetable oils and offer more entrées that are broiled or grilled rather than fried, breaded or sauced. They also offer a greater variety of vegetables, salads and fish dishes than in the past. All of these changes in the food culture make it easier to dine out the green-light way. Here are my top 10 suggestions for not going astray.

1. Just before you go out, have a small bowl of high-fibre, green-light cold cereal (such as All-Bran) with skimmed milk and sweetener. I often add a couple of spoonfuls of no-fat/no-sugar fruit yogurt. This will take the edge off your appetite and get some fibre into your digestive system, which will help reduce the Gi of your upcoming meal.
2. Once seated in the restaurant, drink a glass of water. It will help you feel fuller. A glass of red wine is a good idea too, but wait till the main course arrives before drinking.
3. Once the basket of rolls or bread has been passed round the table – which you will ignore – ask the server to remove it. The longer it sits there, the more tempted you will be to dig in.
4. Order a soup or salad first and tell the server you would like this as soon as possible. This will keep you from sitting there hungry while others are filling up on the bread. For soups, go for vegetable- or bean-based, the chunkier the better. Avoid any that are cream-based, such as vichyssoise. For salads, the golden rule is to keep the dressing on the side. Then you can use a fraction of what the restaurant would normally pour over the greens – and please avoid Caesar salads, which come pre-dressed and often pack as many calories as a burger.

5. Since you probably won't get boiled new potatoes and can't be sure of what type of rice is being served, ask for double vegetables instead. I have yet to find a restaurant that won't oblige.
6. Stick with low-fat cuts of meat (see page 243) or poultry. If necessary, you can remove the skin. Duck is too high in fat. Fish and shellfish are excellent choices but shouldn't be breaded or battered. Tempura is more fat and flour than filling. And remember that servings tend to be generous in restaurants, so eat only 115–175g (4–6oz) (a pack of cards) and leave the rest.
7. As with salads, ask for any sauces to be put on the side.
8. For dessert, fresh fruit and berries, if available, are your best choice – without the ice cream. Most other choices are a dietary disaster. My advice is to avoid dessert. If a birthday cake is being passed around, share your piece with someone. A couple of forkfuls or so along with your coffee should get you off the hook, with minimal dietary damage!
9. Only order decaffeinated coffee. Skim-milk decaf cappuccino is our family's favourite choice.
10. Finally, and perhaps most important, eat slowly. The stomach can take up to half an hour to let the brain know it feels full. So if you eat quickly, you may be shovelling in more food than you require, till the brain finally says stop. You will also be able to savour your meal longer.

SNACKS

RED	YELLOW	GREEN
Muffins (branded)	Popcorn (light, microwaveable)	Fruit yoghurt (fat- free with sweetener
Biscuits	Bananas	Food bars*
Crisps	Most nuts**	Cottage cheese (low-fat or fat-free)
Doughnuts	Ice-cream (low fat)	Almonds**
Ice-cream	Dark chocolate (60–70% cocoa)	Hazelnuts**
Savoury crackers	Raisins	Most fresh fruit
French fries		Most fresh vegetables
Pretzels		Tinned peaches or pears in juice or water
Popcorn (regular microwave)		Ice-cream (low-fat and no added sugar)
Rice cakes		Crispbreads, high-fibre*
Tortilla chips		
Jellies (all varieties)		
Dried fruit and nut mix		
Sweets		

**Warning: Most so-called nutrition bars are high-Gi and high-calorie, with a lot of quick-fix carbs. Look for 50–65g bars, around 200 calories, with 20–30g carbohydrates, 12–15g protein and 5g fat per bar e.g. Myoplex/Slim-fast.*

***6–10 nuts per serving*

SNACKS

Three snacks a day – mid-morning, mid-afternoon and before bed – will keep your digestive system busy, and your energy up. Try to eat a balanced snack, for example a piece of fruit with a few nuts or cottage cheese with celery sticks.

If you're on the move, another convenient snack is half an energy bar. However, most of them are full of cereal and sugar. The ones to look for – Myoplex and Slimfast bars are two examples – are more balanced, listing 20–30g carb, 12–15g protein and 5g fat. *Read the labels carefully.*

Many snacks and desserts are labelled 'low-fat' or 'sugar-free', but they aren't necessarily green-light. Sugar-free instant puddings or 'low-fat' muffins are still high-Gi because they contain highly processed grains.

Dear Rick
Really this email is just a gloat! I have never managed to stick to a diet longer than three or four weeks, and have always felt terribly hard-done-by on them. However, I have now been on the Gi Diet for eight weeks, and I feel great. I started at 11 1/2 stone and am now 10, and if I do say so myself, I look the best I have since I was an awful lot younger! This diet has not only changed my eating habits, but has improved my self-confidence greatly. Eating the Gi way is so easy, and in fact I struggle to eat three meals and three snacks a day as I feel so satisfied with the portions I do eat. I've managed to convert my mother and best friend to the Gi way, not by lecturing them, but just by shrinking every time I se them without any perceived effort!
Heather

BEVERAGES

Because liquids don't trip our satiety mechanisms, it's a waste to take in calories through them. And many beverages are high-calorie. Fruit juice, for example, is a processed product and has a much higher Gi than the fruit or vegetable it is made from. A glass of orange juice contains nearly two and a half times the calories of a fresh orange! So eat the fruit or vegetable rather than drink its juice. That way you'll get all the benefits of its nutrients and fibre while consuming fewer calories.

As well, we should stay away from any beverage that contains added sugar or caffeine. As I explained earlier, caffeine stimulates insulin, which leads to us feeling hungry. So, no coffee or soft drinks containing caffeine in Phase I.

That said, fluids are an important part of any diet and I'm sure you're familiar with the eight-glasses-a-day prescription. The following are your best green-light choices:

WATER

The cheapest, easiest and best thing to drink is plain water. Seventy percent of our body consists of water, which is needed for digestion, circulation, regulation of body temperature, lubrication of joints and healthy skin. We can live for months without food, but we can only survive a few days without water.

Don't feel you have to drink eight glasses of water a day in addition to other beverages. Milk, tea and soft drinks all contribute to the eight-glass-a-day recommendation. But do try to drink a glass of water before each meal – it will help you feel fuller so that you don't overeat.

SKIMMED MILK

After a sceptical start, I've grown to really enjoy skimmed milk, and I like to drink it with breakfast and lunch, which tends to be a little short in protein.

SOFT DRINKS

If you're used to drinking soft drinks, you can still enjoy them if you buy sugar-free diet drinks, preferably caffeine-free ones. People often treat soft drinks or fruit juices as non-foods, but this is how extra calories slip by us.

TEA

Tea has only about one-third of the caffeine of coffee, and it has health benefits as well. Black and green teas contain antioxidant properties that help prevent heart disease and Alzheimer's. In fact, tea has more flavonoids (antioxidants) than any vegetable tested. Two cups of black or green tea have the same amount of antioxidants as seven cups of orange juice or 28 cups of apple juice.

So tea in moderation is fine – minus the sugar and milk, of course. Try different varieties – Darjeeling, Earl Grey, English Breakfast or the spicy chai teas (with sweetener). Herbal teas are also an option, although they lack the flavonoids.

Iced tea is also acceptable if it's sugar-free.

ALCOHOL

I won't bore you with the upside of alcohol, which most of us know; the fact is that it's a disaster if you're concerned about your weight. It puts your blood sugar on a roller coaster: you go up and feel great, then come down and start feeling like having another drink, or eating the whole bowl of peanuts. This cycle of highs and lows can play havoc with your weight-loss programme.

On the other hand, a little red wine can be beneficial for your heart health and, in Phase II, we encourage you to have a glass of wine with dinner. So you can look forward to that. But in the meantime, put away the corkscrew and the ice cube tray because Phase I is a no-alcohol zone.

SUMMARY

- In Phase I, eat only green-light foods – three meals and three balanced snacks per day.
- Drink plenty of fluids, including a 240ml (8fl oz) glass of water with meals and snacks (but no caffeine or alcohol).
- Pay attention to portion size: palm of your hand for protein, and a quarter plate for pasta, potatoes or rice. Use common sense and eat moderate amounts.
- Don't get discouraged by lapses. If you eat green-light 90% of the time, you'll still be fine.

5 Frequently asked questions

Q. How is the Gi Diet different from the Atkins Diet? Can I switch from Atkins to the Gi Diet without gaining weight?

A. The difference is like night and day. The Atkins diet is based on high protein, including animal fat (saturated fat) and very low consumption of carbohydrates. The idea is that when the body is deprived of carbohydrates as the primary source of energy, it will be forced to break down fat instead. The process is called ketosis and, over time, it can cause serious long-term health issues, such as osteoporosis and kidney damage. The high saturated fat content of the Atkins diet is also associated with a higher risk of heart disease, stroke, Alzheimer's and colon and prostate cancers.

Yes, you will probably lose weight on the Atkins diet. But many people gain it all back again, and this yo-yo effect tends to make it even harder to lose weight and keep it off the next time you embark on a diet.

The Gi Diet is just the reverse. Carbohydrates such as fruit, vegetables, whole grains, beans and low-fat dairy products are all encouraged, not limited, while saturated fat is virtually eliminated. If there is one thing that all the health, medical and nutritional authorities agree upon, it is that a diet rich in vegetables, fruits, nuts, legumes, lean meat/fish and whole grains is essential for long-term good health. And that's the Gi Diet in a nutshell.

As high-protein diets are diuretic, you will likely gain some temporary weight when you switch to the Gi Diet and your body rehydrates. When things settle down after a couple of weeks, you will resume your weight loss, while giving your body the nutrition it needs for long-term health.

Q. Is this a good diet for people with diabetes?

A. The key to controlling diabetes is to control blood sugar levels. It is the instability of blood sugar levels and the person's inability to produce enough insulin to remove the sugar from the bloodstream that creates the medical condition called hyperglycaemia. If left uncontrolled, this can lead to death. The glycaemic index was originally developed by Dr David Jenkins to address the issue of which carbohydrates people with diabetes could eat to minimise hyperglycaemia (high blood sugar levels). This is why they find the Gi Diet so effective in the management of their disease. Many have been able to reduce their medications and, in some cases, even eliminate them. As being overweight is one of the key reasons people develop diabetes in the first place, losing weight with the Gi Diet provides a further added benefit.

Q. Will the Gi Diet work for vegetarians?

A. The Gi Diet is an excellent way for vegetarians to eat. Simply replace meat, chicken and fish with alternative protein sources: beans, nuts and soy products such as tofu or tempeh (made from soy beans). The Gi Diet's emphasis on fruits, vegetables, legumes, nuts and low-fat dairy ensures that most nutritional needs are met in spades. A multivitamin is advisable to ensure sufficient B vitamins, which are principally found in meats. (For more on vegetarians' and vegans' nutritional needs, see page 150.)

Q. I seem to have hit a plateau. What should I do?

A. This is a common complaint. The thing to remember is that you never lose weight in a straight line. It drops in a series of short plateaus. You may reach a point for a week or even two or three weeks when your weight doesn't budge. Sound familiar?

As we mentioned earlier, the average weight loss target is 450g (1lb) per week, if you have approximately 10% of your body weight to lose. Count the number of weeks you have been eating the low-Gi way and divide them into the number of pounds lost. This will give you your average weekly weight loss, which you will find almost invariably hits your objective of 450g (1lb) per week. This means you're on target and your weight loss will kick in again soon.

If you are falling behind on your average or the plateau lasts more than a couple of weeks, then you need to check the serving sizes of your green-light foods. Look specifically at serving sizes on the particular green-light products that have been specified, such as potatoes, pasta, rice and nuts (see page 25). Check that you are following the guidelines.

With all other low-Gi products, make sure moderation is your motto. Consuming a 500g tub of low-fat yogurt at a sitting or eating 12 apples a day is clearly not moderation. Be honest with yourself and review what you are currently eating. Keep a food diary for a few days. The only person you are kidding is yourself!

Q. How is the Gi Diet different from the South Beach Diet?

A. Broadly speaking, there are many similarities between the approach taken in the South Beach Diet and the Gi Diet. But there are a couple of significant differences. First, the South Beach Diet has one extra stage; its Phase I is a kind of crash diet. The Gi Diet does not require or recommend a crash diet. Second, the Gi Diet is simpler and easier to use than the South Beach Diet. All the calculations have been done for you. Simply follow the colour-coded charts.

Q. Is it true that the Gi Diet can help relieve depression?
A. While the Gi Diet cannot claim to relieve clinical depression, it can alleviate one of the key compounding factors: blood sugar levels.

Q. What if I fall off the wagon?
A. This is everyone's major concern, and it doesn't need to be. If you can be on the programme for 90% of the time, that's just fine. The worst that can happen is that you will delay reaching your weight target by a week or two. This is a real-world way of eating that recognises the realities of hectic schedules and social pressures of eating on the run and of the sheer temptation to binge on occasion. Again, as with food cravings, the Gi plan has a built-in warning signal whenever you go off the rails. After a few weeks of eating the low-Gi way and keeping your blood sugar levels steady, your body will react with alarm to any sudden onslaught of high-Gi foods. You will end up feeling bloated, tired and irritable. Believe me, it will be a relief to climb back on board the green-light wagon.

Q. Aren't aspartame and other sugar substitutes bad for your health?
A. A great deal of misinformation has been spread about sugar substitutes – driven mainly by the sugar lobby. All the major government and health agencies worldwide have approved the use of sweeteners and sugar substitutes, and not a single peer-reviewed (scholarly) study has identified any health risks. For those who are still concerned about the safety of artificial sweeteners, Diabetes UK has information on sweetners and sugar substitutes on its website (www.diabetes.org.uk) and

there is a comprehensive rundown on sugar substitutes in the US Food and Drug Administration's newsletter, called *FDA Consumer* (see www.fda.gov). If you're sensitive to aspartame, check out such alternatives as sucralose (Splenda®), which is our personal favourite.

Q. Why aren't certain low-calorie foods such as rice cakes or sugar-free jellies green-light?
A. Although they don't have a lot of calories, they are digested quickly, leaving you looking for more food to keep your digestive system busy. The whole idea behind the Gi Diet is to eat low-Gi foods that keep you feeling full for longer, i.e. that are more satiating. Try to stick to green-light snacks, which are far more nutritious and satisfying.

Q. Is the Gi Diet suitable for people who do extended workouts?
A. Absolutely. Other than ensuring your serving sizes are delivering sufficient calories to meet your higher calorie needs, the only modification is the need to replenish your glycogen levels (the body's short-term glucose storage for muscles), which can get depleted during a prolonged workout. Following your workout with a sugar-based sports drink is ideal. Otherwise you may feel lethargic.

Q. I have to travel a lot for business – how can I stay on track with the Gi Diet?
A. Follow the green-light guidlines for eating out on pages 66-71 and 80-82. On planes vegetarian meals are often fresher and more green-light than the standard entrées, which tend to be served with sauces. Call ahead to book them, or bring along your

own supply of almonds, a nutrition bar, a small tub of yogurt or some fruit so that you won't be tempted by the pretzels and cookies handed out mid-flight.

Airports are nutritional deserts, but usually you can scout the cafeterias for a bit of fruit. Some airports now have juice and smoothie concessions. Basically, try to schedule your meals so that you never find yourself hungry in an airport. You'll save money this way, too.

6 Phase II

Well, you've made it. Congratulations! You've hit your target weight, you're digging out clothes you thought you'd never get into again, and you're finally on good terms with your full-length mirror. I hope you are relishing the new you and making the most of your increased energy. Now that you've graduated from Phase I, you can ease up a bit on limiting portion and serving sizes and start adding some yellow-light foods to your diet. The idea here is to get comfortable with your Gi programme; this is how you're going to eat for the rest of your life.

Of course, Phase II is also the danger zone, the stage when most diets go off the rails. Most people think that when they reach their weight-loss goal, they can just drop the diet and go back to their old eating habits. And frankly, when I take a close look at what many of these diets expect you to live on, I can understand why people can't stick to them for long.

The reality is that with some modifications, this is your diet for life. But this isn't a hardship, because the Gi Diet was designed to give you a huge range of healthy choices, so you won't feel hungry, bored or unsatisfied. By now, you will know how to navigate your green-light way around the supermarket aisles, you will know how to decipher food labels, and the colour coding of foods will be second nature. But the strangest thing may be that you are not even tempted to revert to your old ways. If you should fall prey to a double cheeseburger, you will be dismayed at how heavy, sluggish and ungratified you feel afterwards. You will be too attached to your new lightness and levels of energy to abandon them.

Dear Rick
I purposely waited a year before writing to you because I wanted to be sure that this was really a sustainable change in eating patterns. I can now confirm that the Gi Diet is totally sustainable; in fact, I feel more satisfied and less hungry than ever. I cannot conceive of going back to my old ways of eating and do not have the slightest desire to do so. My wife feels the same way. My blood pressure is lower, I no longer have any heartburn, and my workouts are fantastic and fun.
Thanks
Michael

But before we look at some of the new options open to you in Phase II, a word of caution. Your body can now function on less food than before you started. Why? Because you're lighter now, and so your body requires fewer calories. Also, your metabolism has become more efficient, and your body has learned to do more with fewer calories than in its old spendthrift days. Keep these two developments in mind when you head into Phase II. Your eyes may indeed be bigger than your stomach.

So add a few more calories, but don't go berserk. Try not to make a significant shift in your portion/servings, and remember to make yellow-light foods the exception rather than the rule. This way you will keep the balance between the calories you're consuming and the calories you're expending – and that is the secret to stable weight.

As you modestly increase portions of foods that you particularly enjoy and include some yellow-light items as a treat, keep monitoring your weight weekly, and simply adjust your servings up or down until your weight stays stable. This may take several weeks of experimentation. When you've reached the magic balance and can stay there comfortably, that's the formula for the rest of your days. (Give or take a piece of wedding cake or a birthday indulgence.)

Here are some ideas for how you could alter the way you eat in Phase II:

BREAKFAST

- Increase cereal serving size. For instance, go from 50g (2oz) to 75g (3oz) oatmeal.
- Add a slice of 100% whole grain toast and a pat of margarine.
- Double the amount of sliced almonds on your cereal.
- Enjoy an extra slice of back bacon.
- Have a glass of juice now and then.
- Add one of the yellow-light fruits – a banana or apricots – to your cereal.
- And you can now go caffeinated in the coffee department, if you like. But try to keep it to one cup a day.

LUNCH

I suggest you continue to eat lunch as you did in Phase I. This is the one meal that already contained some compromises in the weight-loss portion of the programme.

DINNER

- Add another boiled new potato.
- Increase the rice or pasta serving: rice from 50g (2oz) to 75g (3oz), pasta from 40g (1 1/2oz) to 60g (2 1/2oz) uncooked.
- As a special treat, have a 175g (6oz) steak instead of a 100g (4oz) one.
- Eat a few more olives and nuts (but only a few – these are calorie heavyweights!)
- Try a cob of sweetcorn with a dab of margarine.
- Add a slice of high-fibre bread or crispbread.
- Enjoy a lean cut of lamb or pork.

SNACKS

- Try microwave popcorn (light only), maximum 1/3 packet.
- Increase your serving size of nuts to 10–12.
- Enjoy a square or two of 70% dark chocolate (see below).
- Eat a banana.
- Indulge in one scoop of low-fat ice cream or frozen yogurt.

CHOCOLATE

For many of us, to live without chocolate is not to live. The good news is that in the Gi Diet world, some chocolate – the right sort of chocolate, in the right amounts – is acceptable. I'm sure you've heard that chocolate, like red wine, contains natural elements that help keep the arteries clear. But that is probably not your main motive for eating it; the fact is that chocolate combines fat, sugar and cocoa, all three of which please the palate. However, most chocolate contains too much saturated fat and sugar, which keeps it deep in the red-light zone. Chocolate with a high cocoa content (70% or more) delivers more chocolate intensity per ounce, which means that even a square or two can give chocoholics the fix they need.

ALCOHOL

The other good news in Phase II is that medical research now indicates that a glass of wine with your dinner can help reduce your risk of heart disease and stroke. Red wine, which is rich in flavonoids, is particularly recommended. This requires discipline, though. Just because one glass is beneficial, it doesn't mean that two or three is even better for you. Immoderate drinking undoes any health benefits, and alcohol is always calorific. One glass of wine (150ml [5fl oz] max) provides the optimum benefit.

Apart from red wine, keep your consumption of alcohol to a minimum. I realise that this can be difficult, since drinking is so often a part of social occasions and celebrations. An occasional lapse won't do a lot of harm. But there are various strategies for getting around the social pressure to drink: you can graciously accept that glass of wine or cocktail, raise it in a toast, take a sip, and then discreetly leave it on the nearest buffet table. Faced with a tray of vodka martinis and glasses of red wine, stick with the wine, which lasts longer. My wife, Ruth, drinks spritzers (wine mixed with soda water) on special occasions. And if you add lots of ice to your spritzer, you can reduce the alcohol even further while still joining in the party spirit. Whatever strategy you choose, always try to eat some food with your drink, even if it has to be a forbidden piece of cheese. The fat will slow down the absorption of the alcohol and minimise its impact. (Of course, better to gravitate to the vegetable tray, but an emergency canapé won't be the ruin of you.)

MOTIVATION

The way you look, the response of your family and friends, and the way you feel will all help motivate you to keep on the path. Going back to your old eating habits will seem less like a temptation than a way to undermine all the good things that weight loss has brought you so far. But if your resolve does begin to waver then here are a couple of 'cures' you can try:

THE £5 CURE

This is the food version of what immigrants to Canada (which I am) used to call the '$1,000 Cure'. Whenever a new arrival, after a long cold winter in Canada, started to pine for 'the old country', the cure was to get on a plane and go home for a week. All the reasons that originally persuaded the person to emigrate would come crashing back, until the thought of flying back to Canada began to look pretty good again. (With inflation, this might be more like the '$2,000 Cure'!)

But with food, the cure costs less – say, £5. When you pine for 'the old food', try this: go out for lunch with some friends and order a high-Gi meal – a slice of deep-pan pizza, a beer and a piece of apple pie. Your mouth may enjoy it, but I guarantee that a couple hours later you'll be desperate for a nap, feeling lethargic and lousy. And that's not even factoring in your guilt. Trust me, you won't want to repeat the experience!

SHOPPING BAG TEST

This is an amazing motivator. Fill up a plastic shopping bag – or two if necessary – with some books (your former diet books will work well!) or food tins. Step on the scales and keep adding books or tins until you reach your original weight. Then simply walk up and down the stairs a few times. You'll be so glad that this weight is something you can put down. No wonder you were low on energy and your back and joints ached.

One reader wrote to say that she had lost 32kg (70lb) and tried the Shopping Bag Test. She had to fill four bags, and they were so heavy she couldn't even pick them up. And that was what she had been carrying around all the time. Point taken, she said.

Of course, the Gi Diet is not, and shouldn't be, a straitjacket. Absolute rigidity is the road to disappointment. Try to live 90% within the guidelines of the diet. The idea that certain foods are completely and forever forbidden is bound to drive you, sooner or later, back into their clutches. With the Gi Diet, you are in control of what you eat, and that includes (with discipline, moderation and common sense) almost everything.

SUMMARY

- Use moderation and common sense in adjusting portions and servings.
- Follow the rules at least 90% of the time. Occasional lapses shouldn't be an excuse for giving up entirely.
- For motivation, try the Shopping Bag Test or the £5 Cure.

The Family

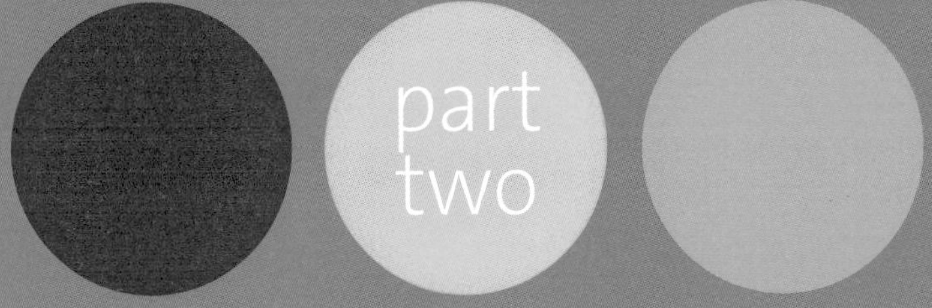

7 The special nutritional needs of women

I have asked my wife, Ruth, to author this chapter to provide a woman's perspective. Ruth is Professor Emeritus at the University of Toronto with a special interest in women's health.

Most of the readers who email Rick about their experiences with the Gi Diet are women. This is hardly surprising given the relationship between popular culture, women's body image, weight and food. But aside from all the sociological reasons why women are so concerned about their weight, the issue of eating will always be more complicated for women because of our physiology, namely the fact that we can bear children. The beginning of our reproductive life, the onset of menstruation and the end, menopause, bring hormonal changes which result in nutritional and weight control concerns. And of course, many women never experience any weight problems until after pregnancy. Let's look at each specific dietary issue in turn.

WOMEN'S METABOLISM

We've had a number of emails from women who tell us about their frustration when their husbands join them on the Gi Diet. They report that the men lose weight faster than they do. Yes, this can happen – and it can be discouraging!

It's not that men are stricter or more disciplined. The reality is that men and women have different metabolisms, and this affects the rate at which our bodies turn food into fuel. Women also have more body fat than men; that's what accounts for our curves. In general, women have about 27% body fat, compared with an average of 15% in men. Men also have more muscle tissue than women, and muscle burns more calories than fat. (That's why your husband can fall off the diet now and then and not pay the price, whereas one piece of birthday cake seems to show up the next morning on your scales.)

Why do women have this extra padding of fat? It plays a role in the natural processes of ovulation, menstruation and reproduction. Fat helps the production and circulation of oestrogen, and ensures that a pregnant woman has some reserves of energy to nourish new life. A woman's body is always, on some level, operating with the potential to sustain another life, even if conception or reproduction never occurs. But what works so beautifully for child-bearing may be counterproductive for trying to lose weight.

Hormones play a huge role in weight control and cravings at different stages of your life. They can affect what you want to eat during pregnancy, and when the levels shift once again during the menopause, hormones can affect blood sugar levels and play havoc with weight control. Then there is the issue of appetite changes affected by PMS (see below). This goes along with a temporary spike in weight (and feeling bloated) that some women experience premenstrually. There are days when women not only 'feel fat', but their weight truly does fluctuate, even when their eating habits don't.

Ageing affects metabolism as well. Women, on average, gain 4.5kg (10lb) per decade, unless they adjust their eating accordingly. The older you get, the fewer calories your body requires. If you're 68 and can't seem to stop gaining weight, take a look at your portions; you shouldn't be eating the same amount you were eating at the age of 50. (For more on the senior years, turn to Chapter 10.)

HOW DIET AFFECTS MENSTRUATION

The age at which girls begin to menstruate has gradually been coming down. Now girls sometimes get their period at the age of 9 or 10. Although the onset of menstruation officially marks the time when the female body is ready for reproduction, it's important to remember that at this age a girl is still growing, and her body isn't 'finished' yet. Young girls, menstruating or not, continue to need the right nutrition to feed both body and brain. Young girls who become diet-crazy and severely restrict their eating can put their overall development at risk, stressing major organs such as the heart and kidneys (see more on eating disorders on page 146).

It's important for girls to have enough fat (preferably the good kind) in their diet; otherwise menstruation will be delayed or interrupted. At a BMI of less than 18, periods are likely to cease. If a girl's diet is so poor that this happens, it's more than likely that other aspects of health are at risk, too. For instance, during the menstrual years, women need to make sure they get enough iron, to replace what they lose during their periods. Women need one and a half times the daily requirement for iron that men do. This is an essential element of haemoglobin, which helps carry oxygen in our blood. When iron levels are too low, we can develop anaemia, which brings with it fatigue, irritability and pallor.

Women who are pregnant or breastfeeding are particularly at risk for low iron. In the developed world, approximately 10% of women are iron-deficient, and this number rises to about 14% during pregnancy. A recent study from the University of Pennsylvania suggests that even mild iron depletion can affect our concentration and ability to think. After improving their iron levels, women with minor deficiencies raised their scores on tests that evaluated attention, short-term and long-term memory.

Normally, if our diet is a good one, we can get all the iron we need from the foods we eat. Red meats (lean cuts of beef or extra-lean minced beef) are excellent sources, as are eggs. Dark leafy vegetables such as broccoli and spinach also contain some iron and are all green-light foods. Seafood and legumes also have some iron.

Menstruation can also affect appetite, cravings and blood sugar levels. Symptoms, such as a desire for sugar, irritability and mood swings, may show up in the second half of the menstrual cycle, when oestrogen levels drop and progesterone rises. (In the first half, oestrogen dominates and progesterone levels are lower.) Early research into the biochemistry of PMS – which wasn't recognised as a physiological reality until recently – discovered that diet can make a difference in the severity of PMS. Dr Katharine Dalton, a pioneering British researcher in this area, found that a diet that emphasised complex carbohydrates and low-fat foods could diminish problems associated with PMS. She also recommends eating three meals a day and three snacks. In other words, the anti-PMS diet perfectly matches the Gi diet. The scientific rationale for this approach is that this way of eating mitigates extreme spikes in blood sugar levels. Simple sugars that are digested quickly only exacerbate symptoms such as depression or irritability. A chocolate bar or a glass of orange juice becomes what you crave, but it also perpetuates the mood swing cycle. Keeping sugar levels stable is critical to managing mood, headaches and food cravings. Recent research has shown that a diet rich in calcium (1,200mg/day) can help prevent or relieve the severity of PMS. Make sure skimmed milk and low-fat yogurts are part of your Gi Diet.

FOOD, DIETING AND PREGNANCY

We all know that pregnancy is a time when we should pay special attention to our diet and nutrition. But don't forget that diet can also affect fertility and that proper nutrition for your child begins at conception. Don't delay: start eating healthily as soon as you start thinking about getting pregnant.

Since being overweight increases the risk of health problems and complications during pregnancy, if your BMI is 25 or over you would be well advised to try to lose some weight before you get pregnant. At the same time, however, adequate body fat is essential for conception, so a too-low BMI is not ideal either. Too much strenuous exercise can lower body fat to the point where it interferes with your ability to conceive. Don't take this as an excuse to turn into a couch potato, but perhaps delay training for the marathon.

If you're hoping to get pregnant, refrain from smoking and drinking alcohol, which can have devastating negative effects on a baby such as lowering birth weight and possibly causing foetal alcohol syndrome. Research also tells us that woman trying to conceive should be sure to get enough folic acid, 400 micrograms (0.4 milligrams) daily. Folic acid is critical for healthy neural tube development (an early part of normal brain growth), which often occurs in the foetus before a woman even knows she's pregnant.

It goes without saying that you are *supposed* to gain weight during pregnancy – most woman gain 10–14 kg (22–30) pounds. But if you are overweight when you become pregnant, you can safely follow Phase I of the Gi Diet. All the foods normally recommended during pregnancy, such as fresh fruit and vegetables, whole grains, lean meat, fish and low-dairy products, are staples of Phase I. However, if this way of eating is a radical change for you, you should talk to your doctor before embarking on the programme.

If your BMI is in the healthy range, Phase II of the Gi Diet is a healthy way for you to eat during pregnancy. It will provide you and your child with the necessary calories and nutrition and help you avoid gaining too much weight. But there are some additional dietary considerations during this special time:

Fish

Fish is an excellent source of protein and omega-3 fats, which evidence suggests can reduce the risk of premature birth, so be sure to include it in your diet. Unfortunately, some fish – the larger species – have been found to contain high levels of mercury, which can damage your baby's brain. Avoid shark, swordfish, mackerel and fresh and frozen tuna when trying to get pregnant and during the first trimester, and limit these to no more than one serving a month thereafter. Tinned tuna appears to be safe in amounts not exceeding 170g (6oz) a week. And you can safely consume up to 340g (12oz) a week of fish such as fresh, frozen and tinned salmon, halibut, sardines and trout, and seafood such as shrimp, squid and octopus. Just make sure that the fish and seafood you eat are fully cooked to kill any disease-causing bacteria or parasites. This is not the time for that barely seared tuna or raw oysters. Also, avoid smoked fish unless it has been cooked in a dish like a casserole.

Aspartame

Though the sugar substitute aspartame has been approved for use by government regulators, no safety limits have yet been established for pregnant or nursing women. Our advice then is to use it sparingly. We prefer Splenda® (sucralose), which is actually derived from sugar.

Listeriosis

Listeriosis is a form of food poisoning that is especially dangerous during pregnancy, possibly leading to premature delivery or miscarriage. It can be caused by unpasteurised cheeses and other dairy products, packaged luncheon meats and raw and undercooked eggs. So avoid eating unpasteurised dairy products, including soft cheeses such as brie, camembert, Roquefort, feta and goats' cheese – which are only used sparingly as a flavour enhancer on the Gi Diet anyway. If you are eating out, ask whether any unpasteurised cheese has been added to the dishes. Don't eat raw or undercooked eggs and avoid luncheon meats unless they have been heated until hot.

Caffeine

Although research indicates that moderate amounts of caffeine (less than 300 milligrams a day from all sources, including coffee, tea, soft drinks and chocolate) won't harm your baby, caffeine does cross the placenta and some studies have linked it to attention deficit disorder and migraines. Some woman find they naturally go off coffee and tea very early in pregnancy, although this aversion can mysteriously wear off by the late stages, when the appetite for old habits may return. If you absolutely must, limit yourself to one cup a day, or have black or green tea, which have beneficial antioxidants and less caffeine than coffee. If you like herbal tea, be cautious: some herbs are not compatible with pregnancy or nursing. Check labels.

Alcohol

Although Phase II of the Gi Diet allows you to enjoy a glass of red wine with dinner, no safe level of alcohol consumption has been established for pregnancy. It is best, then, to avoid it.

'Eating for Two'

Don't let the notion that you are 'eating for two' become your excuse to double your calories. Your baby will not 'use up' your extra body fat. Eating three low-Gi meals and three snacks a day will keep your glucose levels and energy stable and help to control your appetite. But what happens if you start experiencing cravings? Some women crave sweet (chocolate) while others crave sour (the classic one being pickles). I remember craving strawberries. It's not clear why this happens, but it may have something to do with our bodies trying to fulfil a need for a particular nutrient. Try to identify the flavour you are craving and find a green-light food that will assuage it. For example, if you want something sweet and creamy, try low-fat no sugar added ice cream; if you want something sour, have a dill pickle or a salad with lemon juice sprinkled over it. If it's peanut butter you're desperately hankering for, go ahead and savour one tablespoon a day of the natural kind, which contains only peanuts. If it's chocolate that you want, let one square dissolve in your mouth. Be careful not to overdo it.

DIET AND COMMON CONDITIONS DURING PREGNANCY

Morning Sickness

Morning sickness can be a problem for some women during the first trimester. Often particular foods or strong smells trigger nausea; it might be frying bacon or the smell of chicken noodle soup. You'll know when you experience it! Try to find an eating pattern that works for you. Sometimes it helps to eat a piece of whole wheat toast or a cracker before you get up. Or you may find it easier to start the day with a snack, then have breakfast later. If eating full meals puts you off, you might need to forget about meals and slowly graze all day (but keep track, so you know your total daily intake). Drink fluids slowly or drink between meals. Keep a bottle of water handy throughout the day so you can take small sips and stay hydrated, even when the thought of eating turns your stomach. Water will also keep your kidneys functioning well, minimise constipation and make you feel better.

Morning sickness usually abates by week eleven or twelve. For some unlucky women, however, it can persist throughout the pregnancy. If you are vomiting a lot, you should talk to your doctor, since you may be losing essential nutrients (not to mention feeling awful).

Haemorrhoids

Haemorrhoids are another condition that pregnancy can aggravate. The best way to prevent them is to avoid becoming constipated; eat lots of fibre, vegetables and fresh fruit; and drink plenty of water.

Heartburn

Heartburn can develop during the last trimester, and is usually experienced at night. The baby is growing and your uterus is now pressing against your stomach, demanding space. But there are many tricks to minimise or eliminate heartburn, beginning with avoiding spicy and acidic foods. Tomato sauce, citrus fruits, curries, chocolate and decaf coffee can all trigger heartburn. So can eating too quickly, or feeling stressed.

The key to preventing heartburn at night is to eat an early light dinner and to snack lightly (if at all) after 8 p.m. Unlike during the first trimester, when you may have opted for light breakfasts, this might be the time to front-load your day with a larger breakfast, followed by a normal lunch and a light dinner. Believe it or not, raising the head of your bed an inch or two on blocks, or adding an extra pillow to keep the top of your body elevated, can help as well. It's better to treat heartburn through watching when, what and how much you eat rather than relying on antacids or prescription acid inhibitors.

Weight Loss After Pregnancy

Congratulations, you have a new baby, and a new adventure has begun! Though you will lose weight after giving birth – on average between ten and twenty pounds in the first couple of weeks – many women are dismayed to find that they don't immediately return to their pre-pregnancy weight. Be patient, your body has just undergone nine months of tremendous changes and will need time, as much as nine months, to recover. Your main concern right now should be looking after your health, making sure to eat right and get all the nutrients you, and your baby if you are breast-feeding, need. If you were on

Phase II of the Gi Diet during pregnancy and are breast-feeding, you can continue with it now (see more on this below). If you have decided not to breast-feed, you can start with Phase I. If, however, the Gi Diet represents a major change in your eating habits, let your body recover from the birth for three to four weeks before embarking on it. You can also gradually introduce moderate exercise once your body is up to it.

Breast-feeding

Breast-feeding contributes a great deal to the health of your baby, and most experts recommend you do so for about six months. Research suggests that the longer you breast-feed, the less chances your child will have of developing food allergies, and breast milk seems to offer additional immune-strengthening benefits as well. It is worth noting that women who breast-feed use up the extra body fat gained during pregnancy faster than women who don't.

Many women who are breast-feeding ask whether they can remain on the Gi Diet while they nurse their babies – the answer is yes, they can safely follow Phase II. Be sure to drink enough fluids, and include three to four servings of low- or non-fat dairy products or calcium-fortified low-fat soy milk.

Obviously, the quality of your food will affect the quality of your breast milk. Remember that many foods, as well as medications, nicotine and alcohol, cross into the breast milk, so don't go crazy with the celebratory champagne. Remind your GP that you are nursing if any new medications are prescribed, and avoid taking over-the-counter drugs. You may notice that certain foods – onions and garlic are notorious – will affect the taste of your breast milk, sometimes upsetting your baby's stomach, too.

Fatigue

Feeling exhausted almost seems to be a chronic condition in new mothers. Gone are the days of looking forward to six to eight hours of continuous sleep; soon four hours of uninterrupted sleep will seem like a luxury! If this is your first child, you can count on getting some rest during the day, when the baby sleeps. But if you have a toddler and a newborn, a daytime nap may be out of the question. This means that diet becomes even more critical for maintaining your energy and health, though the demands of a new baby make it hard to think about cooking or preparing food. For the first few weeks, try to have your partner or a relative cook for you or bring home nutritious takeaways. Don't try to be superwoman; hand over the reins and be grateful for any help. Be sure to have adequate protein at each meal and snack. Adequate iron is crucial, too: this is a good time to eat lean red meat and eggs.

Try to resist the urge to reach for convenient red-light foods, such as chocolate bars or shop-bought muffins, when you're hungry. Your blood sugar will go up, then plummet, leaving you feeling even more tired and hungry. Instead, keep some green-light snacks on hand which will help tie you over during the early days, when you have little time for shopping and cooking. Keep a stash of green-light nutrition bars for emergencies.

Although you feel exhausted, try to avoid caffeine, or limit yourself to one cup a day. The first few weeks with a baby can be tough, but things settle down eventually. Enjoy this wonderful phase of parenthood, where everything your baby needs is something you can so easily provide.

Dear Rick,
I can't believe that after two pregnancies, and at the age of 32, I weigh what I did in high school! It's thanks to the Gi Diet! I've tried other diets, but this is the one that has changed the way I eat and exercise for life. It has changed my understanding and relationship with food. Some additional positive side effects: no more headaches, no more hunger pains, no more periodic mood swings and 'blues', no more heartburn, and greatly diminished symptoms of PMS and menstrual discomfort...I read the book, began the Gi Diet and have lost 1½ stone as well as 6 inches around the waist...I have never felt better, more active and more energetic. What a joy to be able to go on long hikes, canoe trips and bike rides with my husband and feel terrific doing it!
Janine

MENOPAUSE

Fast-forward now through years of career, homemaking or child rearing to the next great divide in a woman's life: the menopause. From the first hot flush to the last night sweat, menopause can last from 5–10 years, so buckle your seatbelt – it's a long ride, but not necessarily a rough one. Some women breeze through with no complaints at all. Others have to cope with interrupted sleep, a general 'off' feeling, loss of energy and/or libido, and those annoying hot flushes that come out of nowhere and make you want to open every window in the middle of winter.

I'm not going to delve into the pros and cons of hormone replacement therapy (or herbal supplements) here. But I want to point out that one of the side effects of menopause is a drop in your metabolic rate, which is a result of decreased oestrogen. What this means – and you will probably gain some weight before you figure this out – is that you need fewer calories to maintain your weight. So if you don't cut back on either your portions or high-calorie foods, or increase your exercise, you will probably gain some weight. The worst part is that it all seems to head for the waist, the hips and the thighs. This is because oestrogen and progesterone help us maintain that female shape – slim around the waist, curvy at the hips and breasts. But with the menopause, we start to move closer to the male pattern, acquiring fat around the middle. Sad but true! The drop in oestrogen is also connected to an increased risk for osteoporosis, when the bones thin out and become more fragile (see page 119).

What's to be done? Stick with the Gi Diet, and if you're having trouble losing (or the number on the scale keeps going up), go back to Phase I until you arrive at some weight stability. And keep a food diary: it might be that all the life changes involved in the menopause have resulted in some subtle compensation in the food department – more snacks, new treats, bigger portions. Time to keep track of what you really eat and do what you can to cut back on the high-calorie items. And perhaps the best insurance against being buffeted by the menopause is to find some exercise you enjoy and can stick with on a regular basis; try swimming, walking, pilates, t'ai chi, yoga or just getting off the bus or tube a couple of stops earlier on your way to work. The key is consistency, not intensity.

HOT FLUSHES/NIGHT SWEATS

'Is it just me or is it hot in here?' When you're peeling off your sweater and everyone around you is bundled up, you're probably having one of those surges in your internal thermostat that goes along with menopause. During the day, hot flushes are merely annoying, but at night, accompanied by copious sweating, they can interfere with REM sleep and leave you feeling exhausted, even after a full night's sleep. The sweats and flushes are the result of radical shifts in your levels of oestrogen and progesterone, as your body changes gear from the ready-for-reproduction state to a more stable, less cyclical state. Some small adjustments to your diet can help alleviate these symptoms.

- Keep spicy foods to a minimum, especially in the evening.
- Avoid alcohol and caffeine. Alcohol can suppress REM sleep, and caffeine is not only a stimulant but also increases your urge to urinate, and you don't need the added pressure of having to get up for the bathroom!

The Gi Diet is designed to sustain us through all the phases of our life. Women who become family caretakers often forget their own health in their focus on the needs of others. But we need to take care of ourselves for our own sake, first of all, and also for the sake of the people who may depend on us.

WOMEN'S HEALTH CONCERNS

Although we'll be dealing with family health in Chapter 11, we'll address a few conditions here that especially affect women. Although women live longer, we also log more trips to the doctor, and experience more pain and more chronic conditions. So men and women look for different kinds of support from nutrition.

OSTEOPOROSIS

This is a condition that generally concerns women past the menopause, when the decline in oestrogen affects the density of the bones. Women also have smaller bones than men, so this makes us more vulnerable to fragility and fractures. Since oestrogen does affect bone strength, many women are tempted to try, or to stay on, hormone replacement therapy (HRT) for the sake of their bones. But since recent research has emerged pointing out the disadvantages of HRT for many women, these risks (a slightly elevated risk of heart disease, stroke and breast cancer) must be weighed against your individual risk for osteoporosis. There are also other medications that are effective ways to treat osteoporosis.

The most significant degree of bone density loss occurs in the first 2 years after the menopause, so this is when it is absolutely critical that you maintain the calcium levels described below. Bone density tests every couple of years after the age of fifty allow women to monitor how their bone density levels fluctuate. When bones lose density, they become porous and lacy, and fracture more easily. If an ordinary fall results in a broken wrist or ankle, be sure to check your bone density levels.

Although the Gi Diet will go a long way towards delivering all the calcium you require, you should consider adding a daily multivitamin in order to the meet the 1,500 mg level for postmenopausal women. Your supplement should also include vitamin D, which is necessary for the absorption of calcium. This vitamin has to be added to foods (including milk, orange juice and soy milk), or acquired from sunshine. But in northern countries, you can't always count on sunshine delivering enough!

If you are lactose-intolerant, shop for lactose-free items, or take lactase enzyme to help with the digestion of dairy products. If that's still a problem, rely on a calcium supplement with vitamin D to meet your requirements.

The other strategy for beating osteoporosis is to make sure you do regular weight-bearing exercise, such as walking, or working out with small weights. You need to work your bones! Weight-bearing exercise is also all-round good exercise for your heart and your weight management. And walking is free (unless, of course, you want to invest in a pricey pair of walking shoes, which is a good motivator). If your knees give you trouble or your arches are flat, you might look into orthotics, which give arch support and take some of the pressure off overtaxed knees.

BREAST CANCER

Most of us know someone touched by this disease – a sister, a mother, a friend. Or perhaps you have been one of the unlucky one out of nine women who develops breast cancer. The key risk factors include having a mother or sister with breast cancer, early onset of menstruation, or a late first pregnancy. But it can also strike for no clear reason at all. Regardless of your risk factors, diet can play a role in protecting you against breast cancer.

Recent research has shown that being overweight can increase your chances of developing breast cancer. If you are postmenopausal and overweight, you are at a 30% greater risk; if your BMI is in the obesity range, your risk is twice what it is for people of normal weight. It also appears that saturated (bad) fats raise your risk, too. Studies of women living in Japan who get only 10–15% of their diet from animal fats (i.e. saturated fats) show that they have significantly lower rates of breast cancer than in the UK, but when Japanese women move to North America and switch to a typical North American diet, their breast cancer rates change too, becoming the same as other North American women.

Excess alcohol consumption has also been linked to an increased risk of breast cancer, so the Gi Diet will help you cut back on that front, too.

POLYCYSTIC OVARY SYNDROME (PCOS)

Between 5 and 10% of women will be diagnosed with polycystic ovary syndrome sometime during their reproductive years. PCOS is a condition associated with insulin resistance, which leads to hyperinsulinaemia and often obesity. What this means is that the body's ability to get the sugar out of the blood is defective; the cells are unusually 'resistant' to insulin. The pancreas must then secrete more and more insulin to get the sugar out of the blood and into the cells. These high levels of insulin wreak havoc in the body, causing polycystic ovaries, weight gain or difficulty losing weight, increased risk of heart disease and, by the age of 40, up to a 40% increase in the risk of type 2 diabetes or lack of glucose tolerance.

Dear Rick,
I'm eating food I love and still losing weight. All my family have been eating the Gi Diet way, even though I'm the only one who has to lose weight. I suffer from Polycystic Ovarian Syndrome (PCOS), which increases insulin resistance, making it harder to lose weight. So the results I'm having are even better. I never thought I would lose the weight this easily.
Emma

There is no scientific evidence at this time to say that one specific diet is significantly better than another for PCOS, although studies are underway. But there is some evidence that diets promoting stable blood sugar levels are helpful. As a result, many physicians recommend low-glycaemic programmes like the Gi Diet, which is a good choice for anyone at risk for type 2 diabetes.

DEPRESSION

Clinical depression is a multifaceted disorder, often requiring specific treatment. Often it is genetically determined, passing from one generation to the next. However, between feeling good about ourselves and being clinically depressed lies a whole range of feelings. We often describe ourselves as feeling 'depressed' or 'down', and this is where diet, and specifically the Gi Diet, can be helpful. While the Gi Diet cannot cure clinical depression, it may help relieve some of the symptoms.

The Gi Diet helps by stabilising blood sugar levels, and we know this helps stabilise mood. When a person is depressed, blood levels of the mood-regulating neurotransmitter serotonin are lower than normal. Carbohydrates temporarily raise serotonin levels, which is why we reach for high-Gi, simple-carb 'comfort foods' such as doughnuts, bagels and cookies. As we know, simple carbs boost our blood sugar levels quickly, and just as quickly they fall again, and so does our mood. Complex carbs help stabilise our serotonin levels and mood without spiking our blood sugar levels.

Being overweight can be depressing and bad for self-esteem. Attempting diets and failing can often add to these feelings of depression. And with so many fad diets out there promising miracles, failure is almost inevitable. The Gi Diet may produce a less dramatic rate of weight loss, but the weight is more likely to stay off. As so many of our readers tell us, self-confidence and feeling good accompany that permanent weight loss.

Finally, research has shown that regular exercise can relieve symptoms of depression – another reason to put on those sneakers and get walking.

SUMMARY

Women need:

- enough iron to make up for loss through menstruation;
- an 'anti-PMS' diet that promotes stable blood sugar levels;
- sufficient body fat to ensure a healthy reproductive system;
- enough calcium for child-bearing and to inhibit the development of osteoporosis after menopause;
- careful attention to diet during pregnancy and breastfeeding to sustain a healthy baby;
- a diet low in saturated fat
- a low glycaemic index diet.

8 Getting your partner on board

Let's say you live with someone who is indifferent to diets and perfectly happy with how the family eats. But you aren't. You may want to lose weight yourself, and you don't want to do double duty in the kitchen; you may be concerned about your partner's weight more than your own; or you might want your partner to help you turn the children's eating habits around. How do you get your unmotivated partner to go along with the Gi Diet?

First, see if your partner wants to – or should – lose weight. As over half the population is overweight, chances are he or she has a pound or two to lose. In the last chapter Ruth talked about the issues specific to women. Now lets look at the issues that are specific to men.

Men have more **muscle mass** than women, and muscle burns a lot of calories. As we mentioned earlier, we all start to lose muscle mass after our 20s. This process accelerates after 40 in women, and for men it steps up after 60. But since men's total muscle loss is greater than it is for women, this has more influence on their weight, because they're using far fewer calories than when they were younger. For men, this is what suddenly puts the weight on in middle age. Also, with careers peaking and more family obligations, men may not be playing sports or exercising as much as they did when they were younger.

A second factor is **alcohol**. Men drink twice as much as women, and there are three times as many heavy drinkers among men than women. Alcohol is packed with calories and sits at the top of the Gi red-light charts. 'Beer belly' says it all.

The third factor is **body image**. Men simply don't obsess about this in the same way many women do. Being a few pounds up or down – or even many pounds – doesn't necessarily concern them. We all know big, out-of-shape men who don't feel their sex appeal is compromised in the least. Women, on the other hand, can become slaves to body image, never satisfied with their weight or how they look. Whether men are masters of denial or simply lack a woman's finely tuned body awareness, it certainly makes it easier for them to ignore diet and nutrition issues. So if they aren't driven by a desire to get back into their 34-inch trousers, what is going to motivate them to join you on the Gi Diet?

Well, fear of dying might get their attention. If your partner really needs to lose some weight, enlist his doctor's help. Let a doctor tell him about the connection between excess weight and diabetes, heart disease, stroke and cancer. Does he know the link between the saturated fats in porterhouse steaks and the health of his prostate? Is he aware of the association between weight, hypertension and dying of a stroke? If vanity isn't the main issue with many men in terms of losing weight, fear of ill health or of dropping dead at 58 of a heart attack might work.

Males appear to be at greater risk than women for heart disease, stroke and colon cancer. These are all major killers among men. Prostate cancer now kills nearly the same number of men as breast cancer does women. All these conditions are significantly affected by weight and the nature of your diet.

Now get out the tape measure. If your husband's waist measurement is more than 40 inches, he is putting his health in jeopardy. Does he want to miss seeing his children growing up? Do you want to lose your mate and carry the burden of family alone? OK, these are nasty scare tactics, but they are also based on medical reality.

Besides, men want to feel slim and look young too, even if they don't wring their hands about it the way women do. And as soon as they see (and feel) the benefits of losing weight, they won't have to be convinced.

But what if giving up the after-work beer is unthinkable? What if his mother brought him up on giant portions of lasagne and he can't imagine life without it? Scolding and bossing, as you may have discovered, doesn't work with food. The best way to change your partner's eating habits is to stock the house with green-light foods and to provide appealing green-light alternatives to his red-light regulars. Here are some of the recipes in this book that turn traditional meals into green-light ones: Open-Faced Meatball Subs, Mushroom and Gravy Pork Chops, Chicken Fried Rice and Apple Raspberry Coffee Cake.

Once your partner realises that the Gi Diet isn't just 'rabbit food' and deprivation, that he can eat often, lose weight and not go hungry, you may be surprised at how easily he'll be converted. If he notices that he feels more energetic and that the after-dinner slump has disappeared, he'll realise that this way of eating delivers rewards, both short term and long term.

However, perhaps you live with a hard-core objector. He'll eat tuna salad at home, then grab a burger and chips on the way to the football game. Or he'll go along with the food part as long as he can keep up the beer and wine.

There are two routes available in this case. One is to leave him alone. You take the Gi Diet route and let your partner watch your transformation into a slimmer, more energetic, healthier person. Let him notice people noticing how good you look. Once he sees the rewards of the diet – physical and social – he may feel more like joining you.

On the other hand, you can always try the stealth method. Don't try a hard sell. Simply change the family's menu and say nothing. A friend of mine who went on the Gi Diet began serving herself and her husband green-light meals for dinner every night, without telling him they were Gi. He wasn't aware he was on a weight-loss programme until he had to buy a new belt!

If you and your partner are raising kids, he should be aware of what example he's setting: is it the Homer Simpson Diet (I'll have twice what he's having) or an attitude towards food that includes weight control, good nutrition, enjoyment of eating and prevention of disease?

If you are a divorced Dad sharing the parental duties with your ex, don't succumb to the stereotype of the fast-food Dad dining in restaurants with his weekend brood. Show your kids that eating together, preparing meals together and making dinner a family occasion is not going to stop. Don't say you love them with endless treats. Show them you care about them by caring for them, through their diet and nutrition. The Gi Diet is a simple way to organise your single-parent game plan. All you have to do is follow the traffic-light charts.

SUMMARY

Having your spouse/partner involved is important because:

- It makes shopping and food preparation easier.
- It provides you with mutual support and encouragement.
- It represents a cohesive and united front as role models for the family.
- Even if weight loss is not an issue, health will improve through eating better.

9 Are your kids eating well?

Food and children: it couldn't be more important, and it couldn't be more emotionally charged as well. What your children eat has an impact on every aspect of their lives: behaviour, mood, energy, concentration, performance in school and vulnerability to infection and disease. Food is also a source of pleasure and at the centre of family gatherings and celebrations. It's a popular source of conflict, too! Getting a handle on mealtimes is often half the battle in making the whole family run smoothly.

Food also plays an important role in managing medical disorders, including allergies, asthma (which can be related to food allergies) and ADHD, or attention deficit hyperactivity disorder. ADHD affects about 4% of the population and has been linked to childhood obesity. Drugs have been the first line of treatment, but changes in diet can also help enormously.

Then there is the weight issue. About 28% of children in the UK aged 2–10 years old are overweight and obesity rates have tripled in the last 10 years for 6–15 year olds. As health reporter Andre Picard wrote in the *Globe and Mail* (May 2005) on the subject of this shocking modern epidemic of overweight kids: 'Children do not want to be fat. When they are, they pay a terrible price. For the most part, they are voiceless in this discussion and powerless victims of an underlying phenomenon. Overweight and obese children are the product of modern society, one that is characterised by an environment where we have engineered activity out of daily life and adopted a lifestyle that has seen us transform our food into a chemical smorgasbord of fats and sugars wolfed down on the run.'

How do we begin to address all these concerns? The Gi Diet offers one way to turn your family eating habits around. Rich in fruit, vegetables, whole grains, low-fat dairy products and meat, nuts and legumes, the Gi Diet is ideal for growing children. In this chapter, we'll explore ways to involve your children in eating the green-light way, and how to adapt the diet to children with a weight problem, whether they are over- or underweight.

I should add that this chapter does not apply to children under 2 1/2 years; they have specific nutritional needs. For guidelines about feeding your baby, consult your doctor.

THE GI DIET AND CHILDREN

Changing what your family eats is easier said than done! What if your children are perfectly happy living in the no-vegetable zone, on a diet of pizza pockets, supermarket dinners and chocolate? You are probably going to meet some resistance as you try to steer the family meals in a healthier direction. Kids are conservative in their appetites. All the love and goodwill in the world are sometimes not enough to get a 10-year-old to try grilled halibut with mango salsa for the first time. And pushing a new approach to food is often complicated by family dynamics, which tend to play out during mealtimes. This can create tension around who eats what and how much. As many parents have learned, eating is also the area where children can first express their autonomy, and exert control – by spitting out that broccoli or clamping their mouths shut. So it's all too easy for food to become a nasty power issue, with parents and kids on opposite teams.

Mothers especially can invest too much emotion in what their children eat: to feed them, after all, is to love them. To love them even more is to give them more food. Treats can become a way to compensate for not having enough time to spend with your kids. As a result of all these emotional currents, mealtime can be fraught with good intentions and bad eating behaviour.

So as the parent, remember that you are the pivotal factor in how and what your children eat. More often than not, it's up to the mother to decide what everyone in the family eats at home. But it's not just about making the right sort of grocery list; it's also about the attitude that you and your partner share – or don't share – towards food choices, weight, body image and eating. Food is so personal! Perhaps your husband grew up in a family that believed no dinner was complete without 225 or 280g (8 or 10oz) of red meat and a rich dessert. Maybe you had a strict father who made you sit at the table until the last butter bean on your plate was eaten. Now, to your horror, you find yourself doing exactly the same thing with your own child: using food as punishment. Or you might react to too many food rules by doing the opposite with your own children: setting no boundaries at all when it comes to food.

As parents, we need to be vigilant that we are not passing on the poor eating behaviours and attitudes towards weight that we may have grown up with. These only increase the chances of our children developing eating disorders or their own problems with weight control. Where food is concerned, the sins of the father (and mother) are truly visited on their children. These cycles must be broken if we want to do something about the wave of childhood obesity in the culture. The first and simplest way to change, however, is not to add new rules but to lighten up around food. Don't try to overmanage or control how much or what your child eats. Instead, learn to trust your child. Believe it or not, children *will* eat and are quite capable of regulating their food intake. They want to survive after all. And their bodies are good at telling them what they need to survive.

Yes, they might refuse to try new foods at first; this aversion stems from primitive times, when experimenting with new foods or unknown plants could turn out to be fatal. Reassure them that tofu is not, in fact, going to kill them. But don't force it on them. Instead, make new food choices part of mealtimes, so they can experiment or not. Make something different for yourself and let them see you enjoying it. What's important is the kind of 'food environment' you create for them in the home – keeping nutritious things handy and getting rid of the junk food. Then let your children come round to new foods in their own good time. In fact, the more you try to cajole or force food on children, the more likely they are to develop a resistance to eating.

Pushing food is one problem; refusing to let them have any of their favourite foods is another fast route to failure. Too many restrictions in the home may make children overeat when they're out with their friends. So give up on total control. Step back, relax, focus on positive parenting instead, and take a good look at your own eating habits first.

Are you a yo-yo dieter, swinging from a few weeks of rigid rules to an anything-goes attitude? Are you an 'emotional eater', taking comfort in double-fudge ice cream at the end of a bad day? Is your husband a breakfast skipper or a crisps-and-TV-snacker? If yes, then you can't expect your son to sit beside the two of you with a dish of carrot sticks and a wholemeal cracker. The way you relate to food yourself will have the greatest impact on your children's relationship to food. To change them, you have to change yourself as well.

The basic framework governing the relationships between you, your child and food depends on clearly defined roles and responsibilities for both parent and child. Ellyn Satter, in her excellent book *How to Get Your Kid to Eat...but Not Too Much*, suggests a simple formula to prevent food from becoming a battleground:

1. You are the role model who is responsible for *providing meals*, as well as *when* and *where* they will be served.
2. Your children are responsible for *what* and *how much* they eat.

In other words, it's what you do, not what you say, that counts. If you doubt this, think about your mother's feelings around food and ask yourself how it has affected you or your siblings. Maybe she got angry when people were late coming to the table. Do you get upset when people take their time showing up for dinner?

Where do you begin to change your family's eating habits? First of all, if you have been in the habit of catering to different appetites, let your family know that everyone will now be eating the same main meals. And no more grabbing things out of the fridge at all hours. It means that the family will eat together at set times. Maybe not every night at 6 p.m. – lessons, practices and social lives often interfere – but schedule meals in a consistent and regular pattern. For instance, on Monday, Wednesday and Friday, your kids can expect a meal on the table at a certain time and they are expected to be there, too.

It also means that eating together should be a lighthearted time. Keep it enjoyable. This is how we foster a positive attitude towards nutrition and sharing. Don't use meals as an opportunity to raise family problems and conflicts. Not that we're trying to recreate 'Father knows best' here, with the 1950s-style nuclear family – mother in the kitchen, wearing pearls and heels with her dress, and her two well-scrubbed boys sitting at the table. That was probably a fantasy even then! What we are trying to establish is a little *structure* and *predictability* regarding family meals. Believe it or not, most children look for and are grateful for some order and coherence in our uncertain world.

Let's look a little more closely at what's involved if you want to initiate your family into the Gi way of eating.

HOW ARE YOU WITH FOOD?

It's fine to talk the talk – but when it comes to getting your kids to eat more healthily, you have to walk the walk. What, when and how much you eat is going to influence your children much more than a weekly lecture on eating more fresh fruit. Recent research in the USA found that girls who don't like to try new foods are likely to have mums who don't eat a variety of foods, especially vegetables. Try to remember: your grandchildren are probably going to have a few of your eating habits, so make them good ones.

Dear Rick,
My six-year-old son (without any encouragement from me) has begun to change his eating habits after watching what I now eat. Although I am fairly careful with what I feed to him at main meals, his lunchtime sandwich fillings have always been fairly plain and unimaginative (by his choice). But now, for example, he is requesting sandwiches with cucumber, carrot, chicken breast, baby spinach leaves, rocket, tomato and cheese. What's even better is that he makes it himself and takes great pleasure in eating his own creation. So not only has your book changed my life, but it's shaping the future for my son's eating habits as well.
Thank you
Tania

When I was growing up in the UK, we rarely ate fish at home, except for the traditional fried fish and chips, brought home wrapped in a newspaper. So I decided I didn't like fish. When I was raising my own family, my eldest son picked up on this and decided he didn't like fish either. Then I made a conscious effort to change my eating habits and discovered the delights of fresh fish and seafood. We now eat seafood at least twice a week, and our grown-up children have become seafood enthusiasts, too.

A change for the better is welcome, but it also helps to be consistent in what you eat. If you have an all-pizza week, followed by a zero-carb diet week, your children aren't going to listen when you say it's important to drink milk every single day. And children like predictability. They have no problem with the idea that if it's Friday, it's going to be fish. But if your own eating is feast one day, famine the next, or full of guilt over indulging in the 'wrong things', then your children's approach to food will be erratic or fraught with 'issues', too.

Mothers should think twice before they burden their daughters and sons with conversations about being too fat. If you have a thing about your thighs, try not to confide in your 11-year-old daughter about your fixation. Let children feel good about who they are, regardless of what they weigh – and especially if they need to lose weight. The culture is already hard enough on girls and weight without your 'weighing in' with negative remarks that only reinforce this anxiety around having the right sort of curves.

It's more effective to point out the positive results of eating a better diet – the extra energy, the optimism, the social confidence of no longer being overweight, and the feeling of doing the right thing for your body and your health. Don't scare kids into losing weight. It will only backfire in the end.

Don't set up your partner as a bad example either. 'Your father needs to lose weight, so we're all on a diet' is not going to inspire anyone. Kids don't like to hear one parent being disparaged by another. Try to get your partner onside, so he doesn't look down at his Gi plate with its one corner of wholemeal pasta and say, 'That's not real pasta!' If both of you are enthusiastic about eating the green-light way, your kids are already halfway there. You don't want your partner winking at his son and saying, 'Eat your salad, then I'll take you out for a cheeseburger.'

INVOLVING THE FAMILY IN SHOPPING AND PREPARATION

Children are often excluded from food shopping, meal planning and food preparation. There's no reason for this, except that parents are usually rushed and don't want to further complicate their chores. But getting your kids involved in shopping the green-light way is a great strategy for making them feel more in charge of what they eat – and they will learn about nutrition along the way. So engage your kids in this new eating venture. Make it their project, too.

Rather than focus on weight management, talk about this as something that's going to make life better in all kinds of ways – energy, health, appearance, vitality. Explain that it won't be a temporary trial run either. This is how you're going to eat from now on, but don't try to oversell it to your family. You can just consult the traffic-light colour charts, make a list and start shopping.

With your older kids, show them the food charts. You'll be amazed by how quickly they will adopt the traffic-light system and make it part of their language. Many of you will remember the small voice in the back seat telling you to buckle up when seat belts were first made mandatory. This time, it'll be 'Is that chocolate doughnut green-light, Mum?'

If they can read, assign them 'hunting expeditions' in the supermarket: can they find the wholemeal penne? A canned soup with three kinds of beans in it? Which low-fat yogurt is their favourite? Can they find the one with sucrose in it, not aspartame? It's a scavenger hunt for green-light food. Showing kids how to decipher food labels will stand them in good stead for the rest of their lives.

Involve them in the kitchen, too. Our three boys used to help prepare our green-light snacks, such as muffins (see page 227 for the recipe). We have photos of these early muffin makers, complete with their long aprons and large wooden spoons. Children are usually more enthusiastic about what they eat if they helped cook it themselves. Younger children can always wash vegetables, fill measuring cups, stir ingredients or set the table. The older ones can make simple recipes like scrambled eggs, oatmeal cookies and pancakes. Encourage your teenagers to take over the cooking for one family meal a week, if they enjoy working in the kitchen. Let them concoct whatever they want, as long as it fits the green-light guidelines, then give them lots of applause and recognition for a job well done.

Food should be an integral part of family life regardless of what sort of family you have, not just something one parent takes charge of. If your partner doesn't want to cook, ask him to at least play some role in the food department, such as shopping, grilling or growing herbs in the garden. Most men like barbecuing! If you're a single mother, resist the temptation of fast food for you and your kids on your way home from hockey practice. If you're a single father who puts dinner on the table every night, congratulations. Your kids will thank you later (even if they hate the idea of courgettes now).

THE IMPORTANCE OF REGULAR MEALTIMES

When the whole family is on a regular schedule – school, daycare, work, then home again – it's easier to structure mealtimes. But during the summer or on weekends, the whole family can get into all-day snacking and grazing, which is disastrous for weight control and exasperating for the family cook. One minute you're scrambling eggs for the youngest, the next you're putting frozen pizza in the oven for the older ones. Once your children learn that you are willing to cook whatever they want when they want it, you might as well give up!

So set clear, firm times when meals and snacks will be served. If they miss out, too bad. Make a big pot of cooked oatmeal in the morning, and try to make sure everyone sits down to a bowl of it, with fruit and skimmed milk. It takes 5 extra minutes. It might be harder with your teenager. They're notorious for sleeping in, then running out the door and skipping breakfast, or eating a cereal bar on the run. At least make breakfast available to them. Then they might take the 2 minutes to eat it.

If it's summer or the weekend and everyone's in and out of the house, set snack times as well as a dinner hour. At 4 p.m., they can help themselves to the low-fat yogurt or fruit or green-light muffins in the fridge. Otherwise, the fridge stays shut. Grazing all day long encourages high-fat, highly processed, high-calorie choices, and makes it hard to keep track of what you've eaten. So reaching into the fridge for a hunk of cheese is not encouraged. The idea is to sit down together to eat on a regular basis, and at the same time, as often as possible.

THE FAMILY DINNER HOUR

This is an endangered activity. Fewer and fewer families actually sit down together to a cooked meal. Instead, they bring home fast food and eat in front of the TV. This is fun once in a blue moon, but not as a steady diet. Research has shown that people who watch TV while eating tend to overeat. Another familiar scenario is: the family cook prepares a 'kids' meal, then when her partner gets home from work, they sit down to 'adult' food while the kids do homework or watch television.

Eating together not only lets you have more control over nutrition, it fosters many good things: enjoying each other's company, developing manners, conversation and trying new kinds of food. Naturally, people come to the table in all sorts of moods: tired, wound up or angry at a sibling across the table who likes to fight. The dinner table doesn't have to be all peace and harmony, but that time together should be there. Don't talk about family problems. Do that away from the table. Instead, make it a time that is about enjoying the food on the table and each other's company. Younger kids may not want to stay in their chairs too long. Fine. They can manage the main course at least. Just serve a variety of healthy food and let them try it, reject it or simply watch you enjoy it. Exposing them to good food is all you need to do at first.

If possible, create a pleasing environment. Set the table nicely. Turn off the TV, the video games and the mobile phones. Eat slowly. It takes at least 20–30 minutes for the 'I'm full' message to get from stomach to brain.

Again, don't be too rigid around the rules. If there is one night when everyone wants to watch something on TV, at least watch and eat together, and maybe talk about it, too!

Pay attention to the serving portions. In our supersized environment, we tend to offer unnecessarily large portions, even to children. If someone is only 25% of your body weight, don't serve them 75% of your portion. The best solution is to serve foods such as pasta and vegetables in large bowls and have everyone help themselves. Show them how to judge portions by how much of the plate each food covers, remembering that pasta or potatoes should only cover a quarter of the plate and vegetables can fill half the plate. Portions of meat or fish should be the size of the palm of your hand, or a quarter of their (smaller) plate. Serving themselves helps children take charge of what they eat.

Let's look at other ways that children can learn to eat well.

GETTING CHILDREN TO LOVE THE RIGHT KIND OF FOOD

'Just one more bite!' 'Here comes the plane into the hangar.' 'Down the little red lane.' 'Look, I made this especially for you.' Do these sound familiar? My mother's favourite, which she still uses at the age of 95, is 'I love to see an empty plate!' My father liked to 'fly' fingers of toast dipped in egg yolk into the mouths of his grandchildren, with all the appropriate aircraft sounds. And then there's the least effective form of persuasion: 'Remember the starving children in Africa.' How is that supposed to get kids to eat more than they want to?

So cajoling doesn't work, and bribery is not a good idea either. Using treats such as dessert or sweets as a reward only reinforces the appeal of the wrong kind of foods. Forcing children to stay at the table until they've finished what's on the plate is ineffective, too. Associating food with punishment is hardly going to encourage healthy eating habits!

I'M NOT HUNGRY

But if you eliminate coaxing, bribing and scolding, how do you get kids to eat? What if you cook the world's best grilled tuna salad, with green beans and lovely boiled new potatoes, and your child glares at his plate and announces, 'I'm not hungry.' Fine. Let them know they don't have to eat if they don't want to, but they have to stay at the table and keep the family company. Make it clear that you're not going to rustle up something else for them an hour later either. Meals and snacks happen at set times. These are the ground rules. You'll find that hunger is a great motivator. You might also be surprised at how quickly they adapt to a firm schedule around eating.

THE BROCCOLI CHALLENGE

Kids, as I mentioned, don't like to try new things, especially vegetables. Things like kale or Swiss chard or other green veggies often have a slightly bitter taste; in evolutionary terms, people were reluctant to try new things in case they were toxic, and bitterness was often associated with poisonous foods. Breast milk, on the other hand, has a sweetish taste. Perhaps that's one reason why smooth, sweet things appeal to kids so much.

Childhood is about exploring and experimenting, which is what growing up is all about – and that goes for food as well. So be adventurous with nutritious food and with the occasional treats as well. Try low-sugar frozen yogurt. Buy wholemeal raisin biscuits for a change. Explore exotic fruits – star fruit, persimmons, mangoes, papayas. Just as children acquire language skills and reading fluency, they should also develop a knowledge and taste for a wide variety of foods.

Researches claim that it takes 10–15 exposures to a new food before it's fully accepted. If your children don't like the texture of wholemeal pasta compared with the white flour variety, try it again the following week, with a different sauce. They'll get used to it, just as our family got used to skimmed milk instead of semi-skimmed or whole milk.

As for snacks, low-fat yogurts now come in a host of different sizes and flavours, and most kids take to them quickly. Vegetable sticks are great snacks to serve fresh with a yogurt-based dip or hummus. We always kept a plate of sliced or baby carrots, celery sticks and sweet pepper slices in the fridge for the boys. If it's prepared and handy, they will eat it, especially if there aren't any brownies beside them. To this day, veg and dip is a favourite snack in our family.

So the trick to introducing new foods is to offer them without pushing, and to just keep offering them without pushing. I still hate cooked spinach, ever since I was 'obliged' to eat it as a child. Eating should be fun. Make your mealtimes lighthearted; the concrete benefits of weight loss and better nutrition will follow. Encourage kids to develop a sense of accountability and responsibility by making their own choices just as grown-ups do.

Every stage of childhood has different challenges when it comes to diet. Let's look at each of them in more detail.

TODDLER/PRESCHOOL

The years from 2 to 5 are the time when children are most resistant to new foods, especially fresh vegetables. This is when they learn the power of 'no' and of rejecting food.

Some parents find that, if they introduce different kinds of puréed vegetables when first adding solids to their baby's diet, he or she will develop a liking for things like squash, pumpkin, spinach and broccoli. But when a 2-year-old doesn't enjoy the taste of something, he usually lets you know in no uncertain terms! Most of us can remember the first time our toddlers dumped a dish of peas on the floor or spit out a spoonful of egg. Texture is important, too. Sometimes mushed carrots won't appeal, but (when they reach chewing age) carrot sticks with a cup of yogurt for dipping will. Even the shape of the food can make a difference. Celery with hummus in the groove is more fun than plain carrot sticks.

The best way to help your kids open up to new foods is to include them on outings to the supermarket and to restaurants. But let's face facts: as parents of a small child, you are unlikely to spend much time in fancy restaurants. Although advertising and peer pressure is hard to counter, it is possible to raise your toddler to really enjoy fresh vegetables and unprocessed, unpackaged food. It's all a matter of teaching their palette to enjoy different tastes, in the same way you would read to them from many kinds of books or make sure that they visit parks as well as museums. An education in food is as important as any other kind of learning.

FROM 5 TO 12

These are the years when children develop passionate attachments to certain foods and a shuddering revulsion towards others. You will know by now whether your child is a food adventurer or someone who would live only on hot dogs if you let him. I know one boy who grew up in a family of superb cooks, and he was a hot dog aficionado. His mother worried, but eventually he branched out – and he survived.

When kids start school, they are also going to be eating lunch with friends and having sleepovers where a bucket of chicken nuggets is the big draw. The way to balance this school-age romance with fast food and sugary cereals is to stay cool and let it happen; at the same time, make sure what they eat at home is nutritious and varied. Adopt the 75% rule:

The 75% Solution

The golden rule with children, as with adults on the Gi Diet, is not to turn it into a straitjacket. As we wrote earlier, if you keep to the Gi Diet 90% of the time, you'll do well. It's important to give yourself a little leeway for those inevitable situations where you can't control what you eat. Children need more leeway – 75% – to allow for the influence of peer pressure and simple experimentation. Kids don't want to be the only ones bringing a Thermos of bean soup to school, even if they secretly love it. Let them eat what their friends like to eat some of the time. Just keep the home fare green-light and add in yellow-light foods if weight is not an issue. If you can pack green- and yellow-light lunches 75% of the time, you'll be ahead of the game, and your kids won't resent your attitude towards food.

TEENAGE BOYS AND GIRLS

So much goes on between the ages of 12–20: puberty, explosive physical growth, the testing of family bonds and independence, the development of a social network that counts as much (if not more) than the family circle, not to mention the possibility of falling in love and discovering sexual expression. No wonder it's an intense, exasperating and bewildering time for parents as well.

What role does food and diet play in the midst of these roller coaster years? First of all, it provides nutrition for one of the most important stages in your children's physical growth.

Second, it expresses your love for them, even during difficult times. And third, it establishes a relationship with food they will take with them into adulthood. Even when your teenager doesn't want to talk to you about a broken heart, she or he will probably say yes to homemade muffins.

Adolescence is also when food portions either explode or radically shrink. Unfortunately, there is a gender side to all this: teenage boys can develop enormous appetites, while teenage girls, driven by body image concerns, can try to diet in all kinds of unwise ways, which may undermine their nutrition. Your son might think that a mixing bowl full of Cheerios is the answer to his big appetite, but there are other solutions. Your teenage daughter needs to know that not eating is the worst way to lose weight. She'll only gain it right back. Show her yourself that eating more green-light kinds of food will keep her from yo-yoing between extremes of starvation and indulgence. Research indicates that yo-yo dieters end up putting on even more weight than they initially lost! The ideal is slow, steady weight loss or maintaining a stable weight. If your daughter says she wants to lose weight check if her concern is valid by looking up her height and weight on the BMI chart. If her BMI indicates that she is overweight then give her a copy of *The Gi Diet* to read.

Then let her be in charge of selecting the green-light foods she prefers. Make sure she includes good sources of iron, either in food (dark leafy vegetables, for instance) or through a supplement. Menstruating girls need more iron. Help them set reasonable, achievable limits. In order to avoid playing food cop, purge the pantry of tempting red-light items that you or your partner may want to keep around.

Also, remind your kids that everyone is blessed with a

different body type and metabolism, and that there is no universal ideal when it comes to weight.

Unfortunately, adolescence is also a time when eating disorders take hold, especially among teenage girls. The most familiar ones are anorexia nervosa, when they refuse food or eat very little, and bulimia, when they binge on food, then purge through vomiting. Anorexia can be serious, even fatal; when body weight drops below a certain critical point, organs become damaged and can fail. Bulimia can be disastrous to health as well; even teeth enamel suffers from the acidic effect of constant purging. Pay attention to extreme dieting or weight loss in your adolescent daughter. If your daughter is not overweight, then sound nutrition is more valuable than struggling to make it down to size zero.

If, as parents, you are having a rough ride with your adolescent children, one way to offer stability and love is to stick to a regular schedule of family meals and to keep the fridge stocked with green- and yellow-light foods – with room left over for a few totally red-light items that they can't live without. If you can lighten up on the food front while making sure that good food is always handy in the house, you will create an environment that supports and nourishes in every sense.

Skipping meals is common among teenagers. A third of teenage girls, one study estimated, regularly skip breakfast. Since their bodies are in the process of doubling in weight, sleep is at a premium, and sleeping in often becomes more important than sitting down to breakfast in the morning. This starts the domino effect of plunging blood sugar, followed by something sweet to give them energy, and maybe a day of snacks that ends with them overeating at dinner. This is the perfect formula for the classic hyperglycaemic–hypoglycaemic yo-yo, in which they bounce from high to low blood sugar, with the accompanying fatigue and mood swings. Since everything else in their lives is changing so radically, it's a good idea to at least try to keep the blood sugar stable! The skipping-breakfast routine has also been linked to being overweight.

A recent Oxford University study compared two groups of school-age children. One group ate a high-Gi breakfast, the other low-Gi food. At lunch, they were free to choose and eat as much as they wanted. Those on the high-Gi breakfast ate considerably more than those who had the low-Gi fare.

The facts speak for themselves. Practically speaking, how do you convince your headstrong teenager not to bolt out the door with nothing but a chocolate bar in his pocket? Well, if he won't sit down, at least equip him with a green-light-version nutrition bar, in which the fat and sugar content is as low as possible. Better yet, prepare old-fashioned oatmeal for breakfast. Serve it with fruit, almonds, yogurt – whatever strange combinations of green-light toppings he may enjoy. If it's ready when he passes through the kitchen, it will take him 2 minutes to down it, and it will steady his boat for the rest of the day. You might have to get him on the breakfast programme with something more appealing at first, like a fried back-bacon sandwich. But once he compares how he feels on a no-breakfast morning to a day he begins with oatmeal or some other green-light food, he may see the light.

The other way to promote healthy eating and curb peer pressure to eat junk is to encourage your kids to have their friends over and entertain. Mix up your green-light and yellow-light food with their red-light favourites. Let them enjoy offering food and making up their own food combinations. Let food choice become part of their growing independence while you keep the shopping and the meals green-light.

Naturally, the cultural environment plays a big role in our attitudes towards fat and thin as well. Advertising images, rockstars and fashion have a profound influence on how teenagers want to look. Many girls start to smoke as a way to curb weight. And a few will develop eating disorders.

The best way to approach an eating disorder in a teen is with your unconditional support and love, along with good professional help. We may never get to the bottom of the whys of eating disorders, but we can certainly help prevent them by encouraging a relaxed and positive attitude towards eating.

Dear Rick,
As a teenager, I know that dieting is a big thing for a lot of us...we're always trying different diets to try and lose the weight. So many of my friends usually end up going hungry. Because I've witnessed this happen so many times...the idea of dieting completely turned me off, until I found your diet. Considering this was the first diet I've really ever done...I'm surprised that it actually worked. I've been so amazed with the results...I don't want to give away my secret to my friends! I've managed to lose 10kg in a healthy natural way. Even my doctor was pleased with what I had done. And trust me, I'm never hungry!
Erika

VEGETARIANS AND VEGANS

Adolescence is a time when concerns around environmental issues or the treatment of animals can come into play. If your teenager decides to become a vegetarian (eliminating meat from her diet) or a vegan (avoiding all animal products, including eggs and milk), how do you make sure she is getting proper nutrition? How do you shop and cook for a vegan when your husband is a steak lover and your other child won't eat pasta? Well, it's not easy, but it can be done!

VEGETARIANISM

Vegetarian eating is more easily accommodated than veganism, and it has the advantage of emphasising many foods that are green-light anyway: fresh vegetables, whole grains and beans. So vegetarian diets are closer to the Gi Diet than an average diet heavy in processed, sugary or high-fat food. Some teenagers just want to eliminate eating red meat while still enjoying fish, seafood, eggs and other good sources of protein. If this means they will eat more vegetables and whole foods, then the loss of saturated fat in red meat will be a good loss, and protein is not a problem if you include nuts, beans, tofu, soya milk and vegetables in their diet. The only vital nutrient you can't obtain from a diet of plant food alone is vitamin B12, and if your child eats dairy products or eggs, she will get enough B12. What's just as important is iron, but this is available in eggs as well as from dark leafy vegetables. It's important for iron absorption to have vitamin C, so it's a good idea to eat oranges or broccoli with iron-rich foods.

The upside of a vegetarian diet – and it is estimated that up to 35% of teenagers are trying to eliminate red meat from their diet – is the increased awareness of food. If they are concerned about the quality and the origin of what they eat, they will become more aware of other aspects of eating, too. This is better than food oblivion!

VEGANISM

Veganism is a stricter regime, eliminating food from any animal source. So eggs, milk and cheese are out, along with red meat, poultry and seafood. Veganism tends to require more food preparation and careful shopping. This is tougher to integrate into family meals. If your teenager opts for veganism, encourage him or her to get involved in the cooking and preparation of the meals – you will be grateful for the help. But don't be overly concerned about the nutritional deficits of such a diet. A teenager's protein requirement can be completely met by a diet that includes the following elements daily: 90g (3 1/2oz) oatmeal (uncooked), 240ml (8fl oz) soya milk, 2 slices wholemeal bread, 1 bagel, 2 tbsp peanut butter, 200g (7oz) vegetarian baked beans, 140g (5oz) tofu, 2 tbsp almonds, 175g (6oz) broccoli and 250g (9oz) brown rice.

We tend to overestimate our protein requirements and underestimate the amount of protein contained in whole foods such as grains, potatoes and dried beans. The one concern regarding teenagers and vegetarian diets is the overall amount of calories. They need enough calories to maintain their weight, or to lose weight gradually, if that's their goal. So make sure their vegetarian diet is varied. You might need to include certain red- or yellow-light items such as peanut butter, since it's such a popular source of protein; but stick to the all-peanut variety, not sweetened commercial brands.

The only caution with veganism is that this diet does require some form of additional vitamin B12. You can get this from taking nutritional yeast, or from a vitamin supplement.

FAST FOOD AND CHILDREN

The fast-food industry has a lot to account for when it comes to our children's nutrition. Most hamburgers, French fries and other fast-food staples are loaded with saturated fat and calories. Then they made it worse by supersizing everything. You can now buy a 2 litre (72fl oz) Pepsi, but why would you? The book *Fast Food Nation* by Eric Schlosser is an eye opener on the subject. You might also have seen the documentary film *Super Size Me*, by Morgan Spurlock (a book version is available now, too). The film-maker lived on nothing but McDonald's food three times a day for a month, with devastating effects on his weight and health. His doctor finally told him to stop with the Double Quarter Pounders With Cheese if he valued his liver! It's an entertaining portrait that reveals the poverty and perils of a diet dominated by fast food. (And it caused McDonald's to retire the term 'supersize', replacing it with 'large'.)

Let's face facts, however: kids are going to eat fast food from time to time, and your family is going to wind up eating at McDonald's or Burger King now and then. For suggestions on navigating their menus, see the Fast Food section on pages 68–71. With all the red-light temptations, my best advice is to keep family visits to fast-food restaurants to a minimum.

The one exception to the fast-food fat gauntlet is the Subway chain. It provides an excellent range of green-light options, many with less than 7g of fat. Just avoid the Atkins-style wraps, which feature turkey, bacon and sauce; they taste great but are absolutely loaded with saturated fats and calories.

The best solution to eating out is to choose family restaurants.

LUNCHES

This can be tricky. School cafeterias vary from one community to another, and some offer questionable nutritional choices. The only way to have some control over this is to raise your voice and let your school board know your concerns regarding food.

Your other option is to pack a lunch for your children, regardless of how old they are. This chore might be more efficient if you organise your own lunches along with your children's, so only one prep session is required for the whole family. There are tips for turning your child's lunch box into a green-light bag on page 57.

PARTY TIME

This is where you have no choice but to remain flexible. When your children are out of the home and with their friends, they are going to be eating whatever's on the go, which is probably not the healthiest food in the world. Don't be overly critical. You only risk making forbidden foods even more desirable.

Just keep the 75% solution in mind. If they eat green-light at home, they can top up on red-light treats from time to time. They know what's good for them and what isn't. Let them make their own decisions. You're the role model, not the rule enforcer!

IS YOUR CHILD OVERWEIGHT?

While the increase in overweight and obesity statistics among adults has been dramatic, it's even more alarming in the case of children. As I said at the beginning of the chapter, almost 28% of children in the UK aged 2–10 are overweight, and of those 11% are technically obese. The prevalence of obesity is highest in the North East and London.

This is not the place, however, to go into the complex reasons behind the epidemic of childhood obesity. We can blame sedentary habits, video games, and the lack of organized sports activities in school. We can point the finger at TV, and certainly the fast-food and advertising industries have a lot to answer for. We eat more and move less. Recent research suggests that only 3% of adults adhere to the top four behaviours that characterize a healthy lifestyle: maintaining a healthy weight, engaging in regular physical activity, eating more than five servings of fruits and vegetables daily, and not smoking.

Any of those sound familiar to you? Perhaps the best way to address the issue of weight control in your child is to address it in your own life first. However, before you take action, make sure your child really is overweight. Discuss this with your doctor or paediatrician. I have included some charts in Appendix VI that will help you identify whether weight is potentially a problem for your child. But you should then confirm this with your medical adviser.

Let's say your child is definitely overweight and your doctor agrees. The next step is to identify why. Obesity is like a stool with three legs: genetics, diet and exercise. Obviously, we can't do anything about your child's genes. But as parents, we can have a huge impact on the other two factors.

There are steps you can take to help your child lose weight and feel better. As a parent you must:

1. Recognise there is a problem, i.e. that your child is overweight.
2. Recognise that being obese is emotionally and socially hard on your child.
3. Recognise that this is going to affect the long-term health of your child.
4. Recognise that being fat is going to make a difference to your child's performance in school.
5. Recognise that it is your responsibility to help your child.
6. Recognise that what you say is not as important as what you do.
7. Recognise that food cannot become a battleground, because you will lose.
8. Recognise that you need to plan and work with your child, not against him or her. You're on the same team.
9. Recognise that your child is going to need your love, support and optimism to make positive changes.

DIET

There's nothing complicated about the formula for getting fat: if you consume more calories than you expend, you will gain weight. If your child is overweight, he is eating more calories than he burns. Simple. What is more complex is why this should be the case.

When children overeat on a steady basis, there could be many possible contributing factors. Are they unhappy? Bored? Are there family tensions around food, such as arguments and broken rules? Are you a mother whose inability to lose weight causes you to come down hard on other family members who overeat? Or perhaps your child resorts to overeating because of conflict in the marriage that gets acted out at the dinner table. No wonder kids in unhappy households turn to food for comfort.

Eating high-Gi food in particular provides a sugar rush and a temporary lift, and eases the emotional pain. But this soon evaporates, as insulin kicks in and blood sugar levels drop, and soon your 'comfort eater' is looking for his next sugar fix.

One thing you can do for your overweight child is not to single him out. A child with a weight problem is already under intense social pressure from peers and society in general. As a result, he tends to have low self-esteem, poor self-image and frequently suffers from depression, too. The last thing he needs is for you to be on his case.

The answer is to make weight loss a family affair. Introduce everyone, thin or fat, to eating the green-light way. Make it a project you all share and part of a larger focus on family outings or activities, so it's not just about food. If the new diet comes with more weekends spent together enjoying active fun, it will feel like a change for the better, instead of a good-for-you regime.

Try to avoid even using the word 'diet', because this word immediately sets children up for success or failure. Just let them know that you are going to pay more attention to how the whole family eats.

The Gi Diet can accommodate different goals, because family members who are overweight can follow Phase I, while those who don't have to lose weight can expand their food choices and portions by following Phase II, i.e. adding yellow-light foods to their menus.

If both parents are overweight, there is an 80% risk that their children will be overweight. This means that if your children need the Gi Diet, chances are you or your spouse do, too. At least this makes it easier for everyone to get with the programme.

The Gi Diet provides everything your family needs, with its emphasis on the good carbs found in fruits, vegetables, legumes and whole grains; on proteins low in saturated fat, such as turkey, chicken, seafood, lean cuts of meat and low-fat dairy; and on limiting unhealthy saturated fats while promoting polyunsaturated and monounsaturated fats, such as those found in nuts and vegetable oils.

With children, you should increase the amount of good fats in their diet, since these are essential for nourishing growth. You can do this by giving them 100% peanut butter. Although this is a yellow-light food for adults because of its high caloric content, it is a low-Gi food and an excellent source of protein and good fat. But avoid regular and 'light' versions, as some of the peanut content has been replaced with cheaper, unhealthy ingredients, including sugar and starch fillers. All-peanut versions of peanut butter are readily available in supermarkets and health food stores. You need to stir it on opening to keep the oil from separating, but it is the healthiest version.

EXERCISE

This is the third leg of the stool. To control weight, you need to make sure that the amount of calories consumed is not greater than the energy expended. So to tackle a weight problem, you need to focus on a diet that delivers sound nutrition without excess calories, and you need to be active enough to burn off what you eat.

We've lost track of this simple equation. Food is all too ubiquitous, and active fun has a lot of competition from sedentary pleasures like watching TV or playing video games. The multi-channel universe has offered children more reasons for not getting off the sofa. Nowadays, the importance of the internet to schoolwork and the popularity of on-line chatting mean that children and teenagers spend a huge amount of their time moving nothing but their fingers over a keyboard.

Research has shown that children who spend more than 5 hours a day in front of the TV are nearly five times more likely to become overweight than those who watch 2 hours or less. TV watching not only means less activity; it means more eating, in the form of snacks. TV ads aimed at kids don't help either. You don't see many ads selling apples to children.

In many ways, exercise should be 'sold' in the same way that you encourage good nutrition. In other words, it's up to you to get off the couch first and be the role model. So it won't do to have the remote in your hand when you are telling your kids to go play outside for a change. The best way to accomplish this, with younger children at least, is to head off to the nearest park or playground together. Join in on the kids' games. Play football with them. Play tennis with them. Teach the dog to catch a Frisbee.

Bicycling is another activity that kids and adults can enjoy together. If your kids are under 10, stick to bike paths rather than city streets. If you have kids too young to manoeuvre their own bikes, there's a wide variety of bike buggies available, allowing you to pedal while the toddlers get a free and breezy ride. Starting out on the bike paths is also good way to teach kids bike safety rules before they hit the streets. Bicycling also offers you and your family a chance to visit and explore parks and communities outside your neighbourhood. The important thing is to pick a bike frame that fits you, and to adjust the seat so that your leg is extended when the pedal is down. The wrong seat height or too small a bike can put a lot of pressure on the knees.

Are you up for inline skating? If your teenager is into this, you can always accompany him or her on your bike and head for the nearest bike path. Take your cues from your children and their enthusiasms, then find a way to participate if you can. It's easier to try to accommodate their passions rather than ask them to adopt yours. And you might learn something!

Swimming is wonderful exercise, good for both toning muscles and aerobic conditioning. Sign your kids up for swimming classes, and sign yourself up for aquarobics classes, which feature gentle exercises done in a shallow pool. Some gyms even schedule adult classes in one pool at the same time as kids' classes in a training pool. Of course, nothing compares with swimming outside, in a lake or pool. If you're lucky enough to have access to a summer cottage, swimming can be something you enjoy all summer long.

Remember that dancing can be good exercise, too. Lessons in ballroom dancing offer a chance to get aerobic exercise and dress up, too. Exercise doesn't have to be about doing set routines in certain places. Incorporate physical activity of all kinds into your daily life, for the health benefits, for weight loss and just for the sheer pleasure of moving.

Kids just need a nudge to be active. It's what their bodies crave. You'll all be in better moods at the end of a physical day, and you might realise just how dampening TV can be to time spent together as a family. (Then, when you get home from a major expedition on bikes, you can make the rental of a video or DVD a special event, rather than let TV be your regular default position.)

Sports

If you're lucky enough to have an active child involved in aerobic sports, then being overweight should be less of a problem. However, this is one of the few areas where extra dietary care is needed. Demanding sports like long-distance running, soccer and hockey involve a high expenditure of energy over a long period, and can quickly exhaust the glycogen reserves (the short-term medium for readily available glucose, which feeds the muscles). These reserves should be replenished by a sugar-sweetened drink with electrolytes immediately following the activity. Basically, the sport puts you in 'glucose debt', and a sweetened drink helps put you back on track. This is one of the very few times when sugar consumption is a good idea!

SUMMARY

- **Be a role model**. Make your food choices, serving sizes, dining behaviour and exercise habits the kind you want your children to imitate.
- **Be responsible and share responsibility**. You are responsible for providing meals, and for when and where they are served. Your children are responsible for what and how much they eat. If you try to control everything they eat, food will become a battleground, where everyone loses.
- **Make it a family affair**. Don't single out the child who needs to lose the weight. This is not a diet. It's a healthy, nutritious way of eating for the whole family, with the welcome side effect of weight loss for those who aim at that.

10 When I'm sixty-four (or more)

THE GI DIET AND OLDER PEOPLE

If you have an elderly family member living with you, can he or she follow the Gi Diet, too? Should you recommend it to your 78-year-old father, who lives alone and doesn't like to cook? What are the special nutritional needs of elderly people, and how does being overweight differ in its health impact on the elderly? These are all subjects that aren't often addressed by diet books, but if you are over 65 and concerned about your weight, or if you are a caregiver for someone in this stage of life, then these are important questions.

The short answer is yes, the Gi Diet is both healthy and safe for the elderly. While the low-carb, high-fat regimens may strain the heart health of seniors and extremely low-fat diets may even rob them of the nutrients they require to maintain muscle mass and energy, the Gi Diet provides a balance that works well for the changing metabolism and nutritional demands of age.

We are only beginning to learn (and research) how the elderly may differ in the way their bodies process fats and protein. But until we know more, the Gi Diet guarantees a varied range of nutritious food groups and is not confusing to master or follow. The first consideration, as with other age groups, is the risk that obesity poses for those over 65.

One American study has indicated that the number of obese adults over 60 will rise from 14.6 million in 2,000 to 20.9 million in 2010 – a 43% increase. We can anticipate a similar increase in the UK. And the lifetime medical costs for obese men and women will be 42–56% higher than for people of normal weight.

The effect of obesity on the personal health of elderly

people is more costly. Obesity is associated with a greater risk of diabetes, cardiovascular disease, hypertension, stroke, osteoarthritis and some cancers. Furthermore, being overweight restricts the pleasures of physical activity and mobility, and, oddly enough, being overweight doesn't necessarily guarantee sound nutrition either. One study of 2000 older patients by the Geisinger Medical Center in Danville, Pennsylvania, found that over 300 of them were obese, with a BMI of 30 or higher. What was surprising about their nutritional findings was that many overweight and obese older women, especially those living alone, had poor diet quality and didn't get enough fibre, folate, magnesium, iron or zinc, while consuming too much saturated fat. So being fat can co-exist with being undernourished.

Enough of the bad news. There is an upside to getting old. If you make it past 75, you actually become less of a candidate for obesity. And the chances of making it to 75 have improved, too. A hundred years ago, the average life expectancy was 49 years. For women today, it is approaching 80, and for men the mid-70s. Most of you reading this chapter will make it (in one shape or another!) to 85. Whether you feel well and enjoy life at that age will have much to do with your ability to maintain a healthy weight.

As Dr Edward L. Schneider, dean of the school of gerontology at the University of South Carolina, explores in his excellent book, *AgeLess*, the greatest fear around ageing is not death but disability. At 85, half of us will need outside help for bathing, dressing, walking, meal preparation and even going to the toilet. This is not a happy prospect.

What can we do to help prevent this fate? Ill health isn't something we can totally eliminate, but addressing the issue of nutrition in old age, and preventing obesity, can definitely make a difference in how we navigate our senior years. Obesity sets up a domino effect: if you're too heavy to exercise, your bone strength suffers, resulting in a higher risk of fractures if you fall. Limited activity also affects mood and contributes to another scourge of old age: depression. Keeping the pounds off is one of the most effective ways to arm yourself against the slings and arrows of old age.

So we know that being overweight is hard on your body. But new research has also found a direct link between a high BMI and the risk of developing dementia. In a recent issue of *Archives of Internal Medicine*, Swedish researchers found that for subjects with a BMI of 30 or higher, the risk of developing dementia was two and half times greater. If the goal of looking better no longer motivates you at 70, perhaps the hope of thinking better will!

But – and this is the unfair part about ageing – as you get older it only gets harder to shed extra weight. It's not your willpower crumbling; your metabolism and body requirements are shifting. This is a different stage of life, with its own biochemical signature. So let's take a look at why we put on weight as we age.

You may be eating the same and exercising the way you always have (or haven't), and yet after 40, the tape measure turns treacherous. The size 10 trousers go to the back of the closet, and the skirt that used to flatter your hips now doesn't. Your waist feels like a fat-magnet, and if you once enjoyed the classic proportion of 38–28–38, it's more likely to go south and settle on your hips: 38–30–41 is more like it in middle age. (I suppose that's why they call it middle age: that's where all the pounds go!)

Dear Rick
I started on the Gi Diet after seeing the success my daughter had on it. I bought the book and immediately started to lose weight regularly at 2 pounds a week. I am now 65 years old, 5 feet 7 inches tall and have lost over 2 1/2 stone and gone down three dress sizes. At the same time, I have never eaten so well. This isn't like a diet, it just seems to be a healthier way of eating. I am determined to never let myself get fat again as I feel so much better. Before I lost the weight I had constant indigestion and didn't sleep well. Losing weight has, for me, been a great morale booster – I feel so much better about myself.
Pat

So the percentage of body fat goes up and the proportion of lean muscle tissue goes down. In terms of muscle, we peak in our 20s. From then on, it's downhill, as we lose about 2% of our muscle mass with every decade. In middle age, this loss quickly accelerates. For a 40-year-old woman or a 60-year-old man, the loss of muscle increases by 6–8% per decade. Since muscle burns more calories than fat, you're also losing that benefit as well. You're burning up few calories, just when you might be tempted to take in more.

Your energy may not be the same either. You might find you have to do more of the less strenuous forms of activity rather than rely on the high-energy activities you did when you were young. The irony is that, as we age, it's going to take more time and effort to simply maintain our shape, let alone improve it. (And there are increasing arguments to maintain a few extra pounds as we age, as a nutritional buffer and a literal buffer against potential fractures from falls.)

However, if we recalibrate the way we eat, and how much we eat, to reflect the changing metabolism of ageing, it's possible to control our weight and to stay active as well. Both are key to good health and happiness as we age.

Compounding the other factors that put on weight is the tendency to become less active the older we get. For men, active sports like hockey or soccer are replaced by more leisurely ones like golf. Retirement also eliminates the routine activities of the working day. Women who did the physical work of maintaining a household and caring for children may find themselves idling in an empty nest. No more multiple trips up and down the stairs with laundry or chasing after toddlers in the park. The metabolism slows just as our activities begin to slow down as well. (Some studies have found that the metabolic rate can decline as much as 30% over a lifetime.)

So at the age of 70, your body has less muscle, and therefore requires fewer calories. It may use dietary protein less efficiently, and you might also have some digestive issues – heartburn, constipation, irritable bowel syndrome – that discourage you from eating a proper diet. Poor dental health can affect your diet too, not to mention poverty itself, which afflicts the elderly more than any other segment of the population. Depression can dampen the appetite, and so can loneliness. Older widowed men may not have developed kitchen skills, and with age, our sense of taste and smell grow less acute. All of these factors can interfere with eating healthily.

Before we explore how the Gi Diet can help seniors, let's discuss the appropriate BMI for someone over 60. As with children, there are mitigating factors involved. Some extra body fat, as I mentioned above, may help prevent hip fractures in case of a fall. And if you do become seriously ill, the food reserve of a few extra pounds may tide you over during a period when you don't feel like eating. So when you set your BMI target, you may want to aim for the higher side of normal, in the 19 to 25 BMI range. The average for most healthy people is 22. You might want to raise yours to 24–25. This will give you an extra 4.5kg (10lb) or so to draw on in the event of illness. That's not a very comforting rationale for having that extra chunk of dark chocolate, but there is now evidence that people with a slightly higher BMI may live longer. In any case, don't berate yourself if you can't maintain that perfect BMI 22. It might be the wisdom of age at work in your body.

NUTRITIONAL NEEDS

Older people need to pay attention in particular to how much vitamin D, calcium and vitamin B12 that their diet delivers. The body needs more calcium as it ages, to keep the bones strong and to reduce the risk of osteoporosis. Calcium may also help maintain healthy blood pressure and play a role in preventing colon cancer. Elderly people should get about 1,200mg of calcium a day and women 1,500mg, the equivalent of five glasses of milk. You can also get calcium by eating almonds, tinned salmon (with bones), calcium-enriched soy milk or orange juice, and leafy green vegetables such as kale, spinach or Swiss chard.

To make calcium available to the bones, you need vitamin D, which is obtained through exposure to sunlight. Those of us living in northern climes who spend the winters indoors may not get enough sunlight to acquire the recommended amount, 800

IU a day. Also, as we age, the skin's ability to convert sunlight into vitamin D declines. It might take 10 times the exposure to sun for seniors to achieve the same vitamin D levels they had in their youth. Sunscreens can reduce the effect by cutting down the essential UV rays.

Our need for vitamin D doubles after age 50, and triples after age 70. Vitamin D is also important for the prevention of cancer, including breast and colon.

Fortunately, the dairy industry adds vitamin D to all its products, but even on the Gi Diet, which includes low-fat dairy products, you probably won't get enough vitamin D. (Other food sources include deep-sea fish and fish oil – salmon and cod, for instance.) The simplest solution is to take a daily multivitamin as insurance.

To illustrate the importance of this vitamin, consider an American study of seniors' diets conducted, at Tufts University. The group was in the lower half of the normal range of vitamin D levels. Half of them then received a vitamin D supplement, while half took a placebo. The group given vitamin D suffered half as many injuries from falls. This is significant, since falls are the most common form of injury after the age of 65 and are a leading cause of death and disability. Women in particular are vulnerable to hip fractures, and one in five will die as a direct result. So for postmenopausal women, a calcium supplement, in combination with vitamin D, is a good idea.

The other elusive element in old age is vitamin B12. This is essential for heart health and stroke prevention. About a third of older people lack the stomach acid to properly absorb this vitamin from their diet alone, so a separate vitamin B supplement is recommended (the amount in a multivitamin is not enough). Iron deficiency causes 15–30% of anaemia in seniors, but another 10% is caused by B12 deficiency.

Digestion also changes as we get older and we produce fewer digestive enzymes. This means that symptoms such as bloating, indigestion, heartburn and gas become more familiar as we age. We start popping more Tums and thinking twice before eating spicy foods. Christmas can be daunting.

Our bodies normally produce 22 different digestive enzymes, and the foods we eat contain many more. Each enzyme acts on a specific type of food. Protease, for example, helps break down proteins; amylase helps us digest carbohydrates; lipase goes to work on fats, and cellulase, found in plants, helps us digest fibre. This is why products such as lactase enzyme help people who have a problem digesting dairy products and why cellulase helps prevent gas in people who don't process fibre well.

There's no simple answer to this decrease in enzyme production as we age. Taking multiple digestive enzymes won't help since they are mainly destroyed by acids in the stomach. Eating slowly and in a relaxed situation, and chewing thoroughly are probably your best aid to digestion (a glass of red wine might also help).

Since older adults also have a decreased sensation of thirst, it pays to make a habit of taking lots of fluids – water, milk, tea or clear soup. Dehydration can lead to constipation, another nuisance that comes with age.

With this advice in mind, then, following the Gi Diet is an excellent way for seniors to stay on track, both in terms of weight management and optimum health.

Dear Rick
I am a seventy-year-old man and have been on various diets and weight control programmes for most of my life. Until the Gi Diet, each one had limited effect and failed in one way or another. I have now been on the Gi Diet for four months, and have lost approximately 15 kilograms. Never have I felt hungry or deprived. On the contrary, I think I eat more now than before! I have also reduced my waist measurement by 4 inches and weigh less than I did when I joined the RAF at age eighteen! As well, my blood sugar levels are controlled without medication, and my blood pressure and cholesterol are down as well. The renewed energy and feeling of well-being are amazing. I recommend this diet to everyone, even if weight loss is not the prime goal. I will be on this programme for the rest of my life.
Thank you!
Gordon

STAYING ACTIVE

Let's be quite clear about this: if you want to maintain a healthy weight, live longer and prevent disability and dependence in your old age, exercise is not an option, it's a must. But it doesn't have to mean running marathons, lifting dumbbells, or enduring disco-driven aerobics classes. There are all kinds of pleasant, low-key ways to include physical activity in your life.

A few years ago, the advice regarding exercise was 'no pain, no gain'. You had to sweat, sprint, get your heart rate up and push your limit. Recent evidence, however, suggests that any activity is better than none, and that 30 minutes of brisk walking a day can be just as beneficial as more intense workouts. The only problem with exercise for older adults is that the benefits tend to evaporate rather quickly, so you have to be active on a regular basis. In our youth, you could get away with a lapse in activity and the muscles might not even notice. At the age of 70, however, a lazy week will reverse all the hard work you've done maintaining muscle tone – and more important than having shapely calves, you want to sustain an independent lifestyle as long as you can. Other than diet, the single best thing you can do to ensure this is to get off the sofa. The risk of nearly all the 'old-age' diseases – cancer, heart, stroke, diabetes, dementia – are significantly reduced by exercise. Yes, a glass of wine with dinner and a good laugh at a sitcom on TV are good for your health too, but only in combination with daily activity. The secret is to find an exercise you enjoy doing.

There are three areas of exercise that complement one another.

Note: You should talk to your doctor before embarking on an exercise programme in any case.

AEROBIC/CARDIO

Aerobic exercise – going up a flight of stairs is one example – works your heart, lungs and muscles all at once. At the gym, you can get an aerobic workout by swimming, using the treadmill, cross-trainer or stair climber machine. Some machines will even tell you, by combining your weight and age, what your target heart rate should be and when the aerobic benefits kick in. (Also, you don't want to exercise too strenuously for your current state of health.)

You can also work on a stationary bicycle at home, but many elderly people are already socially isolated, so sometimes joining a gym offers not only exercise but also provides more community as well. The YMCA has a number of programmes designed especially for older adults, including aquarobics, where gentle exercises are done in a heated pool. They also offer a degree of subsidy for those who can't afford the fees. Many gyms and health clubs also have all-female facilities, which are popular with older women who don't want to work out in a sea of young athletes.

If you're not the gym type, you can get your aerobic exercise simply by making a habit of walking briskly – as if you were late for an appointment – every day for 30 minutes. If the weather is nasty, try 'mall aerobics': drive to the nearest shopping arcade and walk from one end to the other and back. For the truly enterprising, jogging, biking and cross-country skiing are endurance sports that can be enjoyed into old age. Jackrabbit Johannsen, the famous Norwegian-Canadian cross-country skier, participated in ski marathons well into his 80s and 90s (and lived to be 111!)

STRENGTH TRAINING

This helps you maintain strong bones and keeps your muscles toned. In a gym, ask the staff to make sure that you are using the strength-training equipment properly. Some people assume that pushing heavier weights will get faster results, but you set yourself up for injuries if you do this. The key to strength training is to start small, using lots of repetitions with low weights.

Increase the number of repetitions rather than adding more weights.

At home, use a set of 1, 1 1/2 and 2kg weights. A yoga mat helps with balance and traction. Dyna-Bands – stretchy rubber sashes that you use during exercise to create resistance – are good for gentle strength training, too.

STRETCHING/FLEXIBILITY

Stretching is good for muscles, tendons, ligaments and joints. Also, it helps in the general aches and pains department, making stair climbing and housework easier. Staying flexible also develops your balance and minimises potential injuries from falls.

Why do falls happen? Sometimes, it's as simple as not lifting the front of your foot high enough as you take a step. This can happen when your calf muscles lose flexibility which is particularly the case in women after a lifetime of wearing high heels; you begin to shuffle rather than lift the foot. That makes it easier for you to catch your toe and fall. Needless to say, for women, wearing high heels only adds to the risk.

Osteoporosis is the likely culprit with curved spines, but regular stretching can help combat this tendency. Stretching alone can result in a 100% increase in flexibility in just one week!

Any gym will offer advice on simple stretching exercises, but one of the best ways to stay supple is to join a yoga class. One weekly yoga class can do wonders, not only for lower back pain but also for posture, stress and mood. The emphasis on deep, regular breathing is also nourishing to the muscles and relaxing. Once you learn the ropes in class, yoga exercises are also easy to do at home. You're never too old to enjoy the benefits of this ancient practice.

The exercise system known as pilates is also excellent for older people, because it lets you go at your own speed. Developed by dancers for strengthening the body and dealing with injuries, this technique is as demanding or as gentle as your body requires. It focuses on increasing your core strength, the abdominal and back muscles in particular. It's a wonderful way to prevent or diminish lower back pain, and it has postural benefits as well.

SUMMARY

- The Gi Diet will help you lose weight and keep it off.
- If you improve your health, you'll reduce your risk of falling prey to today's major diseases and disabilities.
- Take a multivitamin to address possible calcium and vitamin D deficiencies. A vitamin B supplement is also recommended.
- Incorporate some aerobic exercise, strength training and stretching into your routine.
- Remember, use it or lose it!

11 How the Family Gi Diet can fight disease

Foods are fuel and a source of pleasure, too, but food can also have a biochemical effect on us that's as powerful as any drug. Everything we eat affects our health, well-being and emotional state, and this happens four or five times a day. Most of the time, we're looking for the pleasure angle rather than biochemistry. Imagine if we went to the medicine cabinet and chose our drugs the same way! The right foods can help you lose and maintain your weight, protect your health, extend your lifespan, give you more energy, and make you feel good and sleep better. Couple that with exercise and you are doing all you can to keep healthy, fit and alert. The rest is a matter of genes and luck.

Let's take a look at how diet acts as a critical factor in preventing some familiar diseases.

HEART DISEASE AND STROKE

These are the two biggies. Heart disease and stroke account for about 40% of all deaths in England and Wales. Nearly half of those who suffer heart attacks are under the age of 65. And the simple fact is that many of those heart attacks could have been prevented by diet.

The more overweight you are, the more likely it is you will suffer a heart attack or stroke. The key factors linking these two diseases to diet are cholesterol and hypertension (high blood pressure). I won't go into the detailed science here. But everyone should understand a little bit about the role and significance of cholesterol and hypertension.

One of the harbingers of both heart attack and stroke is high blood pressure, or hypertension. Think of the circulatory system as a garden hose where the force of the water is too great. With hypertension, there is too much stress on the arterial system, which causes it to age and deteriorate too rapidly. This eventually leads to arterial damage, blood clots and a heart attack or stroke. In simple terms, a blockage in an artery to the heart triggers a heart attack (not enough blood and oxygen reach the heart), and a blockage in an artery going to or in the brain will cause a stroke.

Why are we talking about medical matters in a diet book? Because excess weight has a major bearing on blood pressure, which in turn can trigger these life-threatening consequences. A recent study demonstrated that a lower-fat diet, coupled with sizable increase in fruits and vegetables (eight to ten servings a day) lowered blood pressure. In other words, the Gi Diet is the way to lower your blood pressure and reduce your risk of disease.

As for cholesterol, it has a bad reputation, but we need to understand its role more clearly. Cholesterol itself is essential to your body's metabolism, and we can't live without it, but high levels of cholesterol contribute to the plaque that builds up in your arteries, eventually causing blockage.

To make things more complicated, as you probably know, there are two forms of cholesterol: HDL (the good kind) and LDL (the bad). The idea is to boost HDL while suppressing LDL. (One way to remember the difference: HDL is 'Heart's Delight Level', and LDL is 'Leads to Death Level'.) What pushes the LDL levels up into the danger zone? Saturated fat. The kind that turns solid at room temperature – like the stuff you skim off chicken soup and the lovely white lard you bake into a pie crust. This is also what marbles tasty steak and makes bacon sizzle in the pan. Saturated fat is also present in whole milk and hidden in crackers and pretzels. Not only do polyunsaturated and monounsaturated fats work to lower LDL levels, but they also actually boost HDL. So the no-fat diet is not a good idea. Instead, make sure that the right sort of fat is part of what you eat. (For the full picture on fats, refer to Chapter 1.)

DIABETES

Diabetes is the kissing cousin of heart disease, in the sense that more people die of heart complications arising from having diabetes than from diabetes alone. Diabetes rates are skyrocketing: they are expected to double in the next 10 years.

The most common form of diabetes is called type 2; it used to be called Adult Onset Diabetes as well, but now so many children are developing diabetes that the name had to be changed. The main causes of the alarming rise in type 2 diabetes are obesity and lack of exercise. The fact that we are a culture in love with sugar contributes. 1.8 million people in the UK have the disease and over 150 million world-wide and these figures are increasing at an astonishing rate. It is predicted that, in the UK alone, another 1.2 million people will be diagnosed with diabetes over the next 5 years.

Now diabetics themselves have discovered that eating a low-Gi diet releases sugar more slowly into the bloodstream and helps stabilise blood sugar levels, which, in turn, helps them control their diabetes. It has the additional advantage of helping them lose weight, which is the most common cause of diabetes in the first place.

But prevention of diabetes is preferable to management, and that's where low-Gi eating is really useful.

CANCER

Every year, the evidence mounts that weight and diet are critical risk factors for most forms of cancer. Diets high in animal fats (saturated), such as the low-carb, high-protein regimes that have been popular, are directly associated with increased vulnerability to breast, colon and prostate cancers. On the other hand, people who eat more fresh vegetables, fruits and whole grains seem to have a lower risk of developing these cancers. The American Institute for Cancer Research recommends that people eat a predominantly plant-based diet that includes a variety of vegetables, fruits and grains – in other words, the Gi Diet.

ALZHEIMER'S

Over the past 2–3 years, there has been a steady flow of research studies linking Alzheimer's and dementia to diet. A diet high in saturated fat can double the risk of getting this dreadful disease. As we mentioned earlier, anyone with a BMI of 30 or higher is two and a half times more likely to develop dementia. (Note: This study was based on data from more than 7,000 men. We don't know the implications for women.) Alcohol, salt and refined carbs were also associated with risk.

On the upside, a diet rich in deep-sea fish (i.e. oily fish, such as sardines, mackerel and herring) can help prevent Alzheimer's. It seems that omega-3 oil and the vitamin E found in these fish are the helpful agents. Many studies suggest that the anti-inflammatory effect of antioxidants found in nuts and green vegetables, such as spinach, broccoli and Brussels sprouts, which are also rich in vitamins C and E, may have a protective effect against Alzheimer's.

Well, you know the bottom line here: the Gi Diet is low in saturated fat and rich in omega-3 and vitamin E. It's your best line of defence against the loss of your cognitive abilities and memory in advanced age.

ARTHRITIS

Again diet seems to be very helpful in managing arthritis, especially osteoarthritis. First, being overweight already puts a strain on joints, especially weight-bearing ones. What if your knees, hips and ankles have to absorb an extra 22.5–27kg (50–60lb) of impact every time your foot hits the ground? Try lifting a 22.5kg (50lb) weight and you'll see what your poor body is coping with. Don't make your joints work harder than they have to.

ABDOMINAL FAT

The most alarming medical news about fat, which runs contrary to our popular assumptions, is that it is not a passive accumulator of energy or extra baggage. Rather, it is an active, living part of your body. Once it accumulates enough mass, fat behaves very much like any of the body organs, such as the liver, heart or kidneys. This 'beer belly' organ actively undermines your health by pumping out a dangerous combination of free fatty acids and proteins. This causes rapid cell proliferation, which is associated with the growth of malignant cancer tumours. In other words, fat seems to spur the growth of cancer, when those cells are present.

Fat also creates inflammation, which is linked to atherosclerosis (artery thickening), which in turn causes heart disease and stroke. It also increases insulin resistance, which leads to type 2 diabetes. So a beer belly, or 'apple shape', is not just an inert lump of fat. These tissues behave more like a huge tumour, actively undermining health in other parts of your body. Not a pleasant thought.

PROSTATE HEALTH

Just as a low-fat diet can help protect women from developing breast cancer, a diet low in saturated fat has been shown to offer protection to men from prostate cancer, which is even more pervasive among older men. Eating too much red meat puts men at higher risk of both colon and prostate cancer. A diet low in animal fats and high in fresh fruits and vegetables is a prostate-friendly diet – in other words, the Gi Diet.

Recipes

The Recipes

Notes

- In all recipes 1 tbsp = 3 tsp (15ml)
- In many recipes we use rapeseed oil. If this is unavailable then use a yellow-light vegetable oil.

BREAKFAST

GRANOLA TOPPED PEACHES 

Eating fresh fruit for breakfast gives you a healthy start to the day. In this dish, peaches are combined with granola and cottage cheese for an additional energy boost. They can also be served cold.

50g (1⅔oz) jumbo oats
30g (1oz) almonds, flaked
15g (½ oz) All Bran or 100% bran cereal
6 ripe peaches
1 tbsp soft non-hydrogenated margarine
1 tub (500g/1lb 2oz)) no/low-fat cottage cheese
2 tbsp sugar substitute
45g (1½oz) dried cranberries or raisins
2 tsp orange rind, grated

1. In a non-stick frying pan, toast rolled oats and almonds over medium heat, stirring constantly for about 8 minutes or until golden brown. Place in a bowl. Add bran cereal and set aside.

2. Meanwhile, cut peaches in half horizontally and remove stone. Melt margarine in a large non-stick frying pan over medium heat and place peaches cut side down and cook for about 5 minutes or until starting to soften. Remove to a plate.

3. In a bowl, stir together the cottage cheese, sugar substitute, cranberries and orange rind. Divide evenly among the peach halves. Sprinkle with the oat mixture.

Makes 6 servings.

CANNED PEACH OPTION: You can substitute 12 canned large peach halves, drained, for the fresh peaches. Omit the cooking step 2 for the peaches.
PEAR OPTION: Try using 6 ripe Williams pears for the peaches. Nectarines would also work well.

ORANGE BERRY WAFFLES 

This simple recipe freezes well, so be sure to make extra waffles for weekday breakfasts. A couple of slices of back bacon on the side add protein to the meal.

85g (3oz) wholemeal flour
35g (1¼oz) wheat bran
2 tbsp sugar substitute
¼ tsp cinnamon
Pinch salt
275ml (10fl oz) skimmed milk
2 medium eggs, whisked
1 tsp vanilla
3 egg whites, whisked

Orange Berry Compote
2 oranges, peeled
225g (8oz) sliced strawberries, fresh or frozen
225g (8oz) fresh or frozen blueberries
3 tbsp water
3 tbsp sugar substitute or to taste
2 tbsp cornflour

1. Make the Orange Berry Compote: Chop the oranges, reserving juices, and place in saucepan. Add the strawberries, blueberries, water, sugar substitute and cornflour and bring to the boil, stirring occasionally. Cook for 1 minute or until thickened and remove from heat.

2. In a bowl, whisk together the flour, bran, sugar substitute, cinnamon and salt; set aside. In another bowl, whisk together the milk, egg and vanilla. Pour over the flour mixture and whisk until combined.

3. In another bowl, beat the egg whites until stiff peaks form. Fold into the batter.

4. Heat a waffle iron. Spray lightly with cooking spray and pour in about 8 tbsp of the batter. Close lid and cook for about 4 minutes or until the steam stops and waffle is golden. Serve with sauce. Repeat until all the batter is used.

Makes 6–8 servings.

STORAGE: Waffles can be wrapped individually and frozen for up to 1 month. Reheat in a microwave or, for a crisper waffle, in a toaster. Orange Berry Compote can be refrigerated for up to 2 days and reheated over a low heat or in the microwave.

MINI BREAKFAST PUFFS 

Ideal for those rushed mornings, these muffin-sized puffs are packed with nutrition.

1 tsp rapeseed oil
1 small onion, chopped
1 red pepper, chopped
225g (8oz) chopped broccoli
½ tsp dried thyme
¼ tsp each salt and freshly ground black pepper
85g (3oz) crumbled light feta cheese
7 eggs, whisked
225ml (8fl oz) skimmed milk
12g (¼oz) wheat bran
30g (1oz) wholemeal flour

1. In a non-stick frying pan, heat oil over a medium heat and cook the the onion and pepper for about 5 minutes or until softened. Add broccoli, thyme, salt and pepper; cover and steam for 3 minutes or until the broccoli is tender crisp and bright green. Divide the mixture among 12 greased muffin tins; set aside.

2. Sprinkle the cheese over the top of vegetable mixture.

3. In a bowl, whisk together the eggs, milk, bran and wholemeal flour. Pour evenly over the vegetable and cheese mixture. Bake in the oven at 200°C (400°F; gas mark 6) for about 20 minutes or until golden, set and puffed. Let cool slightly before serving.

Makes 12 puffs (6–8 servings).

STORAGE: These can be made up to 3 days ahead and kept refrigerated and reheated in the microwave for instant breakfasts.
HELPFUL HINT: You can serve the muffins with a salad for a light lunch.
CHEESE OPTION: Try using low fat Cheddar cheese.

HAM AND ASPARAGUS BREAKFAST BREAD 

This bread makes a wonderful addition at brunch. Feel free to substitute the asparagus with other vegetables, such as chopped courgette, seeded chopped tomatoes or roasted red pepper.

175g (6oz) asparagus, chopped
175g (6oz) wholemeal flour
30g (1oz) wheat bran
2 tsp baking powder
¼ tsp salt
180ml (6½fl oz) skimmed milk
3 medium eggs, whisked
55g (2oz) non-hydrogenated soft margarine, melted
115g (4oz) chopped lean ham or back bacon
2 spring onions, chopped

1. In a large non-stick frying pan, bring 110ml (4fl oz) of water to boil; add asparagus. Cover and steam for 3 minutes or until tender crisp and bright green. Drain and rinse with cold water. Drain well; set aside.

2. In a bowl, whisk together the flour, bran, baking powder and salt. In another bowl, whisk together the milk, whisked eggs and margarine. Pour over the flour mixture and stir to combine. Stir in the cooked asparagus, ham and onions until combined.

3. Pour into a greased 23cm (9in) square baking dish and bake in the oven at 190°C (375°F; gas mark 5) for about 25 minutes a knife inserted in the centre comes out clean.

Makes 9 bars.

VEGETARIAN OPTION: Omit the ham and use a vegetable base pepperoni or slice of bacon

EGG AND HAM TORTILLA ROLL UP 

These roll-ups are a favourite breakfast and lunch dish, so make stacks of egg pancakes ahead of time and store them in the fridge.

1 tsp rapeseed oil
1 spring onion, chopped
2 medium eggs, whisked
Pinch each salt and freshly ground black pepper
35g (1¼ oz) cooked red kidney beans
¼ tsp dried oregano
1 small wholemeal tortilla
1 slice lean ham or turkey (optional)

1. In a small non-stick frying pan, heat oil over a medium heat and cook the onion for about 1 minute or until softened.

2. Whisk the eggs, salt and pepper together. Pour into the frying pan and stir using a heat-resistant spatula for about 30 seconds or until the mixture is beginning to set. Cook for about 2 minutes or until the egg is no longer runny.

3. Meanwhile in a bowl, mash the beans and oregano until smooth. Spread over tortilla and top with the ham or turkey slice, if using. Slide the egg pancake on top and roll up.

Makes 1 serving.

CHEESE OPTION: Try sprinkling 2 tbsp light crumbled feta or shredded low fat Cheddar or Swiss cheese over the top before rolling up.
SALSA OPTION: Spread 1 tbsp (15ml) low fat salsa over the top before rolling up.

VEGETABLE FRITTATA

Frittatas are a great way to get your family to eat their veggies. Use whatever vegetables you have in the fridge to create this nutritious breakfast or lunch dish.

2 tsp extra virgin olive oil
1 onion, chopped
2 cloves garlic, finely chopped
1 yellow pepper, chopped
175g (6oz) sliced mushrooms
1 tsp Italian herb seasoning
Pinch hot chilli flakes
140g (5oz) fresh or frozen peas
6 medium eggs, whisked
¼ tsp each salt and freshly ground black pepper

1. In a non-stick frying pan, heat the oil over a medium heat and cook the onion, garlic, pepper, mushrooms, Italian herb seasoning and hot pepper flakes for about 8 minutes or until the liquid has evaporated from the mushrooms. Add peas and cook for a further 2 minutes, stirring constantly.

2. In a bowl, whisk together the whisked eggs, salt and pepper. Pour into the frying pan, stirring well to combine the vegetables and egg mixture. Lift the edge around the frying pan to let the mixture run underneath and cook for about 5 minutes or until the top is not runny and the bottom is golden.

3. Place a plate large enough to cover the frying pan over top and invert pan to remove frittata. Slide frittata back into frying pan and cook for a further 5 minutes or until golden and a knife inserted in centre comes out clean.

Makes 4–6 servings.

HELPFUL HINT: You can serve wedges of frittata open faced on wholemeal bread. Frittatas can be enjoyed hot or cold with a salad.

SOUPS

CHICKEN VEGETABLE NOODLE SOUP 

This soup is the ultimate in comfort food for adults and kids alike. For variety, try it with turkey instead of the chicken.

1 tbsp rapeseed oil
1 leek, white and light green part only, thinly sliced
2 stalks celery, chopped
1 carrot, chopped
4 cloves garlic, finely chopped
225g (8oz) mushrooms, sliced
1 tbsp freshly chopped or 1 tsp dried thyme
½ tsp freshly ground black pepper
¼ tsp salt
1.4 litres (2½ pints) chicken stock (low fat, low sodium)
3 boneless skinless chicken breasts, diced
40g (1½oz) orzo pasta
1 can (410g) red kidney beans, drained and rinsed
225g (8oz) lightly packed shredded spinach

1. In a stockpot heat the oil over a medium heat and cook leeks for about 5 minutes or until beginning to soften. Add the celery, carrot, garlic, mushrooms, thyme, pepper and salt and cook, stirring for about 8 minutes or until the liquid evaporates from the mushrooms and starts to turn golden.

2. Add the chicken stock and bring to boil. Add the chicken and orzo, and cook, stirring occasionally for about 10 minutes or until the chicken is no longer pink inside and the pasta is al dente. Add the spinach and beans and cook until the spinach is wilted and beans are hot.

Makes 6–8 servings.

VEGETARIAN OPTION: To make this soup vegetarian simply substitute vegetable stock and use 400g (14oz) diced firm tofu instead of the chicken.

HEARTY LENTIL TOMATO SOUP 

This isn't your average thin, watery tomato soup. It's packed with vegetables and is rich in flavour. Fill a Thermos for lunch at work or school. For an added kick, sprinkle soup with hot chilli flakes before serving.

2 tsp rapeseed oil
1 large onion, finely chopped
3 cloves garlic, finely chopped
1 carrot, chopped
1 celery stalk, chopped
1 tsp Italian herb seasoning
225g (8oz) dried green lentils
2 tbsp tomato paste
1.4 litres (2½ pints) vegetable stock (low fat, low sodium)
1 can (400g) chopped tomatoes
200g (7oz) diced firm tofu
450g (1lb) fresh or frozen peas
¼ tsp each salt and freshly ground black pepper

1. In a stockpot heat the oil over a medium heat and cook the onion, garlic, carrot, celery and Italian herb seasoning for about 8 minutes or until softened. Add the lentils and tomato paste and cook stirring for 2 minutes. Add the stock and chopped tomatoes and bring to the boil. Cover and reduce heat and boil gently for about 1 hour or until the lentils are tender.

2. Add the tofu, peas, salt and pepper and cook for 5 minutes or until the peas are tender and cooked through.

Makes 4–6 servings.

STORAGE: You can freeze this soup for up to 1 month. Thaw in the refrigerator and reheat in a saucepan or microwave.

BEEF AND KALE SOUP 

Kale is a great source of vitamin C and folate. Combine it with beef to make a hearty soup for cold winter days. The brave can add a dash of hot pepper sauce to their servings.

1 tsp rapeseed oil
1 onion, thinly sliced
2 cloves garlic, finely chopped
½ tsp ground cumin
½ tsp ground coriander
1 litre (2 pints) beef stock (low fat, low sodium)
225g (8oz) kale, finely shredded
1 top sirloin grilling steak (about 225g [8oz])
1 can (410g) red kidney beans, drained and rinsed
Pinch each of salt and freshly ground black pepper

1. In a pot, heat the oil over a medium heat and cook the onion, garlic, cumin and coriander for about 8 minutes or until softened and beginning to get golden. Add the stock and bring to the boil. Add the kale and cook, stirring occasionally for 5 minutes.

2. Meanwhile, trim any fat from the steak and discard. Slice the steak into thin strips and cut the strips in half crosswise. Add to the soup along with the beans, salt and pepper, and cook, stirring occasionally, for about 10 minutes or until the kale is tender and steak is slightly pink inside.

Makes 3–4 servings.

CHICKEN OPTION: You can substitute 2 boneless skinless chicken breasts for the beef, thinly sliced and cooked until no longer pink inside.
SPINACH OPTION: You can substitute spinach or Swiss chard for the kale.
BEAN OPTION: You can substitute cannellini beans, lentils or black beans for the red kidney beans.

SALADS

CHICKPEA AND CHICKEN SALAD 

Chickpeas and chicken make a great combination. This salad can also be served in half a wholemeal pitta with lettuce and tomato slices.

2 tsp rapeseed oil
15g (½oz) freshly chopped flat leaf parsley
½ tsp ground cumin
½ tsp each salt and freshly ground black pepper
2 boneless and skinless chicken breasts
1 can (410g) chickpeas, drained and rinsed
4 sticks celery, chopped
200g (7oz) each red and green pepper, chopped
2 spring onions, chopped
100g (3½oz) shredded Cos or leaf lettuce

225ml (8 fl oz) no/low-fat mayonnaise
3 tbsp plain no/low-fat yogurt
¼ tsp grated lemon rind
1 tbsp lemon juice
2 tsp sugar substitute
½ tsp chilli powder or to taste
1 small clove garlic, finely chopped

1. In a bowl, combine the oil, 2 tbsp of the parsley, cumin and half each of the salt and pepper. Add the chicken and toss to coat evenly. Place breasts on greased grill over medium–high heat and cook for about 10 minutes or until no longer pink inside. Remove to a plate and set aside.

2. In another large bowl, combine the chickpeas, celery, peppers, onions and lettuce.

3. In a small bowl, whisk together the mayonnaise, yogurt, lemon rind and juice, sugar substitute, chilli powder and garlic. Add the remaining parsley, salt and pepper.

4. Pour over the chickpea mixture and stir to combine.

5. Chop chicken into bite size pieces and add to salad. Toss to combine.

Makes 4 servings.

HELPFUL HINT: You can substitute leftover chicken for the chicken breasts.
TURKEY OPTION: You can substitute turkey for the chicken.
TOFU OPTION: You can use 275g (10oz) chopped extra firm tofu (either flavoured or plain).
CUCUMBER OPTION: If you don't want to use red or green peppers, use ½ chopped cucumber.

THREE BEAN SALAD

Packed with fibre, this classic salad is perfect for lunch or a snack. Make extra to refrigerate for another day.

450g (1lb) green beans, trimmed
1 can (410g) red kidney beans, drained and rinsed
1 can (410g) chickpeas, drained and rinsed
4 sticks celery, chopped
1 medium red onion, chopped
75ml (3fl oz) red wine vinegar
2 tbsp extra virgin olive oil
1 clove garlic, finely chopped
1 tbsp Dijon mustard
1 tsp celery seed
¼ tsp each salt and freshly ground black pepper
10g (⅓oz) freshly chopped flat leaf parsley
10g (⅓oz) freshly chopped mint or basil
100g (3½oz) Cos lettuce, torn
100g (3½oz) baby spinach leaves

1. Cut the green and yellow beans into 2.5cm (1in) pieces. Cook beans in a saucepan of boiling salted water for about 7 minutes or until tender crisp. Drain and rinse under cold water until cool. Drain well. Place in a large bowl and add the red kidney beans and chickpeas, celery and onion to bowl.

2. In a small bowl, whisk together the vinegar, oil, garlic, mustard, celery seed, salt and pepper. Pour over the bean mixture with the parsley and basil. Toss to coat evenly.

3. Combine the lettuce and spinach and divide among 4 plates. Divide the bean mixture evenly over the lettuce mixture to serve.

Makes 4–6 servings.

TOFU OPTION: Omit 1 can of the beans and add 275g (10oz) diced extra firm tofu to the salad.

WHEAT BERRY APPLE CRANBERRY SALAD 

Wheat berries are whole wheat kernels and are high in fibre. When mixed with apples and tart cranberries, the result is a definite winner. If you cannot get hold of wheat berries then you can use bulgar wheat instead..

1 cup wheat berries
2 Granny Smith apples, cored and chopped
120g (4oz) baby spinach
1 can (410g) mixed beans, drained and rinsed
90g (3oz) dried cranberries
3 tbsp orange juice
2 tbsp apple cider vinegar
1 tbsp rapeseed oil
1 small clove garlic, finely chopped
2 tsp Dijon mustard
¼ tsp each salt and freshly ground black pepper
15g (½oz) freshly chopped mint or flat leaf parsley

1. In a large pot of boiling water, cook the wheat berries, covered, for about 1 hour or until tender but still slightly chewy. Drain and rinse under cold water until cool. Drain well and place in a large bowl. Add apples, spinach, beans and cranberries.

2. In a small bowl, whisk together orange juice, vinegar, oil, garlic, mustard, salt and pepper. Pour over the wheat berry mixture and toss to coat. Add the mint or parsley and stir to combine well.

Makes 6–8 servings.

TUNA SALAD BOATS

Canned tuna is a good source of protein and easy to prepare. It is also a popular request for lunch, so my advice is to make it interesting and make it often.

115g (4oz) cooked chickpeas
2 cans (120g each) chunk tuna
packed in water, drained
4 sticks celery, chopped
60g (2oz) red pepper, chopped
1 dill pickle, finely chopped
50ml (2fl oz) no/low-fat mayonnaise
2 tbsp plain no/low-fat yogurt
1 tbsp lemon juice
¼ tsp each salt and freshly ground black pepper
4 small leaves butterhead or radicchio lettuce
¼ cucumber, thinly sliced
1 tomato, cut in wedges

1. In a bowl, and using a potato masher, mash the chickpeas coarsely. Add tuna, celery, pepper and pickle.

2. In a small bowl, whisk together the mayonnaise, yogurt, lemon juice, salt and pepper. Scrape this over the tuna mixture and stir to combine well. Divide tuna mixture among lettuce leaves and garnish with cucumber slices and tomato wedges.

Makes 4 servings.

SALMON OPTION: You can substitute 2 cans (213g each) red salmon, drained, for the tuna.
CELERY STALK OPTION: Spoon the tuna salad onto 8 large celery stalks.

VILLAGE SALAD

This is a variation on a classic Greek salad. The addition of beans and hearty greens adds much needed protein and fibre.

200g (7oz) shredded Cos lettuce or chicory
4 tomatoes, cut into thin wedges
1 green pepper, thinly sliced
1 can (410g) cannellini beans, drained and rinsed
85g (3oz) diced light feta cheese
½ cucumber, thinly sliced
55g (2oz) chopped, pitted olives (kalamata are best)
2 tbsp lemon juice
1 tbsp extra virgin olive oil
1 clove garlic, finely chopped
¼ tsp each salt and freshly ground black pepper
2 tbsp each freshly chopped oregano and flat leaf parsley
1 tbsp freshly chopped mint

1. In a large shallow bowl, combine the lettuce, tomatoes, pepper and kidney beans. Top with the feta, cucumber and olives.

2. In a small bowl, whisk together the lemon juice, oil, garlic, salt and pepper. Pour over the salad and toss to coat. Add the oregano, parsley and mint and toss to combine well.

Makes 4–6 servings.

TUNA OPTION: For more flavour, add 2 cans (120 g each) chunk tuna packed in water, drained.

MEATLESS

BEAN TACOS 

Serve these tacos with a variety of toppings, along with basmati rice and salad.

2 tsp rapeseed oil
1 onion, chopped
2 cloves garlic, finely chopped
1 green pepper, chopped
½ tsp chilli powder or to taste
1 tsp paprika
½ tsp ground cumin
2 cans (410g each) red kidney beans, drained and rinsed
225ml (8fl oz) low fat salsa
8 small wholemeal tortillas
90g (3oz) Cos lettuce, shredded
2 tomatoes, chopped
125ml (4fl oz) no/low-fat sour cream

1. In a large non-stick frying pan, heat the oil over a medium heat and cook the onion, garlic, pepper, chilli powder, paprika and cumin for about 5 minutes or until softened.

2. Add the beans and salsa and cook for 5 minutes or until heated through. Using a potato masher, mash about half of the bean mixture. Stir together to combine.

3. Divide the bean mixture among the tortillas and top with lettuce, tomatoes and sour cream.

Makes 4 servings.

BEAN OPTION: You can substitute black beans or cannellini for the red kidney beans.
HELPFUL HINT: You can also serve this up as a salad; simply increase the amount of lettuce and top with the bean mixture. You can drizzle a little vinaigrette on it or squeeze a wedge of lime over before serving.

VEGGIE BEAN BURGER

Fibre-rich bean burgers are easy and inexpensive to make, highly nutritious and delicious.

1 can (410g) cannellini beans or lentils, drained and rinsed
1 egg
30g (1oz) wheat bran
30g (1oz) almonds, finely chopped
2 tbsp freshly chopped mint
1 small clove garlic, finely chopped
¼ tsp each salt and freshly
ground black pepper
2 tsp rapeseed oil

Coriander Yogurt Sauce

50ml (2fl oz) no/low-fat plain yogurt
1 tbsp freshly chopped coriander
¼ tsp ground cumin
Pinch salt

1. In a large bowl, using a potato masher, mash beans until smooth. Stir in the egg, bran, almonds, mint, garlic, salt and pepper until well combined. Divide the mixture into 4 equal portions and form into 1cm (1/2in) thick patties.

2. In a large non-stick frying pan, heat the oil over a medium heat and cook the burgers for about 12 minutes, turning once or until golden brown.

3. Meanwhile, in bowl, stir together the yogurt, coriander, cumin and salt until combined. Dollop onto burgers before serving.

Makes 4 servings.

HELPFUL HINT: These burgers can be served on half a wholemeal bun with sliced tomatoes, cucumbers and lettuce.

ASIAN NOODLE STIR-FRY 

Mung bean noodles can be found in the international aisle of the supermarket. They come in little bundles or one large bundle. It is easiest to weigh the bundles for the correct amount, but each little bundle weighs approximately 40g (1 1/2oz), which means you will need about three small bundles for this recipe.

115g (4oz) mung bean noodles
2 tsp rapeseed oil
1 onion, thinly sliced
1 carrot, thinly sliced
1 aubergine, thinly sliced
1 red or green pepper, thinly sliced
450g (1lb) chopped broccoli
200g (7oz) chopped extra firm tofu
125ml (4fl oz) vegetable stock (low fat, low sodium)
50ml (2fl oz) orange juice
50ml (2fl oz) hoisin sauce
1 tbsp ginger, freshly chopped
½ tsp chilli sauce or hot chilli flakes or to taste
75g (2½oz) chopped roasted cashews

1. In a large bowl, cover the noodles with hot water and let stand for 10 minutes or until softened. Drain and set aside.

2. In a large non-stick frying pan, or wok, heat the oil over a medium–high heat and stir-fry the onion, carrot, aubergine, pepper and broccoli for about 8 minutes or until beginning to get golden and softened. Add the tofu and stir to combine.

3. In a bowl, whisk together the stock, juice, hoisin sauce, ginger and chilli sauce. Add the noodles and sauce into the frying pan and toss to combine; cook for about 3 minutes or until the sauce has coated all the vegetables and the noodles are hot.

Makes 4 servings.

SOUTHWEST VEGGIE BAKE ●

There are many varieties of frozen mixed vegetables on the market, and using them makes this casserole easy to prepare. Look for colourful combinations with an assortment of vegetables, such as Asian mixes with red pepper, green beans and mushrooms.

450ml (16fl oz) low fat salsa
2 medium eggs, whisked
2 tbsp freshly chopped coriander
2 tsp dried oregano
½ tsp ground cumin
Pinch each salt and freshly ground black pepper
340g (12 oz) Quorn mince
1 can (310g) black beans, drained and rinsed
450g (1lb) frozen mixed vegetables
55g (2oz) low fat Cheddar cheese

1. In a bowl, stir together the salsa, egg, coriander, oregano, cumin, salt and pepper. Break up the Quorn mince and add to the salsa mixture with black beans; stir to combine and set aside.

2. Place the vegetables into a greased 20cm (8in) casserole dish. Cover and microwave on High for 5 minutes. Drain any excess water and top with Quorn mince mixture and sprinkle with cheese. Cover with foil and bake in a 200°C (400°F, gas mark 6) oven for about 30 minutes or until hot throughout.

Makes 4–6 servings.

HELPFUL HINT: Bake this mixture into 4 small casseroles, perfect for family members to carry along for lunch the next day.

FISH AND SEAFOOD

BROCCOLI STUFFED SOLE 

These stuffed fish fillets are impressive enough to serve to company. For this recipe, thin fish fillets like sole, tilapia or catfish work best.

1 tsp rapeseed oil
1 shallot, finely chopped
2 cloves garlic, finely chopped
225g (8oz) chopped broccoli
150g (5½oz) cooked red kidney beans, chopped
50ml (2fl oz) fish or vegetable stock or water
50g (2oz) light garlic and herb cream cheese
2 tbsp freshly chopped flat leaf parsley
2 tbsp freshly chopped chives
6 sole fillets, about 20cm (8in) long (about 675g [1½lb] in total)
¼ tsp each salt and freshly ground black pepper

1. In a non-stick frying pan, heat the oil over a medium heat and cook the shallot and garlic for 2 minutes. Add the broccoli, kidney beans and stock. Cover and cook for about 3 minutes or until the broccoli is tender crisp. Stir in the cream cheese, parsley and chives. Let cool slightly.

2. Divide the broccoli mixture crosswise in the centre of the fillets. Roll up gently to cover the filling and place in a small baking pan. Sprinkle with salt and pepper. Bake in an 210° (425°F, gas mark 7) oven for about 15 minutes or until the fish flakes easily when tested with fork.

Makes 4–6 servings.

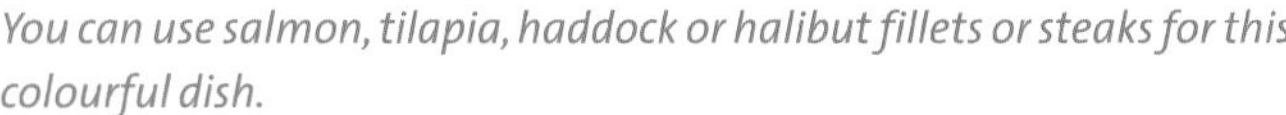

VEGETABLE TOPPED FISH FILLETS

You can use salmon, tilapia, haddock or halibut fillets or steaks for this colourful dish.

2 tsp extra virgin olive oil
450g (1lb) small mushrooms, quartered
1 medium red onion, chopped
2 cloves garlic, finely chopped
About 25 cherry tomatoes, halved
1 courgette, chopped
2 tbsp freshly chopped flat leaf parsley
2 tbsp freshly chopped basil
¼ tsp each salt and freshly ground black pepper
6 fish fillets, about 675g (1½lb) in total
6 lemon wedges

1. In a large non-stick frying pan, heat the oil over a medium–high heat and cook the mushrooms, onion and garlic for about 5 minutes or until beginning to turn golden. Add the tomatoes, courgette, parsley, basil, salt and pepper and cook for about 5 minutes or until the juices begin to form.

2. Meanwhile, place the fish fillets on greaseproof paper-lined baking sheet. Top each fillet with vegetable mixture. Bake in a 210°C (425°F, gas mark 7) oven for about 15 minutes or until the fish flakes easily when tested with fork. Squeeze each piece with lemon wedge before serving.

Makes 6 servings.

MUSHROOM OPTION: Try using a mixture of chopped shitake and oyster mushrooms for a different flavour.

TERIYAKE FISH KEBABS 

These marinated fish kebabs are easy to make and festive. Serve them with basmati rice and steamed baby pak choi.

50ml (2fl oz) soy sauce
1 spring onion, finely chopped
1 tsp finely freshly chopped ginger
1 tsp Dijon mustard
1 small clove garlic, finely chopped
675g (1½lb) halibut fillets, skinned
1 small courgette, halved lengthwise
225g (8oz) small button mushrooms
2 tsp toasted sesame oil
Pinch pepper

1. In a bowl, whisk together the soy sauce, spring onion, ginger, mustard and garlic; set aside. Cut the halibut into 6mm (1½in) pieces and add to the soy mixture. Toss to coat and let marinate for 10 minutes.

2. Meanwhile, cut the courgette into 1cm (½in) pieces and place in a bowl. Add the mushrooms and drizzle with sesame oil and pepper. Toss to coat.

3. Skewer halibut, courgette and mushrooms alternately onto 6 metal or bamboo skewers. Place on a greased grill over a medium–high heat and grill for about 10 minutes turning once or until the fish flakes easily with a fork, and vegetables are tender crisp.

Makes 6 servings.

HELPFUL HINT: If you are using bamboo skewers, you will need to soak them for about 15 minutes in water to help eliminate flare-ups.
YELLOW-LIGHT BEEF OPTION: You can substitute 450g (1lb) top sirloin grilling steak for the fish. Marinate for 15 minutes and grill for about 12 minutes or until cooked.

SALMON CAKES WITH TARRAGON TARTAR SAUCE 

These fish cakes are quick and easy, and a favourite with kids. Serve them alongside asparagus and carrots, or pack them into pittas with lettuce and tomato. Make mini salmon cakes for a great party appetiser.

2 cans (213g) salmon, drained
150g (5½oz) cooked cannellini beans
1 egg
55g (2oz) finely chopped red pepper
2 spring onions, finely chopped
1 small clove garlic, finely chopped
2 tbsp freshly chopped flat leaf parsley
Pinch each salt and freshly
ground black pepper
2 tsp rapeseed oil
Tarragon Tartar Sauce
50ml (2fl oz) no/low-fat mayonnaise
1 tbsp lemon juice
1 tbsp finely chopped dill pickle
2 tsp freshly chopped tarragon
Pinch each salt and freshly ground black pepper
2 wholemeal pitta breads
2 tomatoes, sliced
85g (3fl oz) shredded Cos lettuce

1. In a large bowl, using a potato masher, mash the salmon and beans until combined well. Stir in the egg, red pepper, onions, garlic, parsley, salt and pepper until well combined. Divide mixture into 8 equal portions and form into 1cm(½in) thick patties.

2. In a large non-stick frying pan, heat the oil over a medium heat and cook the salmon cakes for about 10 minutes or until golden brown and crisp.

3. Meanwhile make the sauce: in a bowl, whisk together the mayonnaise, lemon juice, pickle, tarragon, salt and pepper; set aside.

4. Cut the pitta breads in half and open. Divide the tomato and lettuce among the pittas. Fill with salmon cakes and dollop with tartar sauce.

Makes 4 servings.

TUNA CASSEROLE 

This Gi-friendly version of a traditional family favourite uses wholemeal noodles and less cheese.

225g (8oz) wholemeal rotini or fusilli pasta
280g (10oz) frozen mixed vegetables
2 tbsp rapeseed oil
1 medium onion, finely chopped
1 tsp dried thyme
½ tsp dry mustard
30g (1oz) wholemeal flour
450ml (16fl oz) skimmed milk
¼ tsp salt
Pinch pepper
3 cans (120g each) chunk tuna packed in water, drained
2 tbsp grated Parmesan cheese

1. In a large pot of boiling salted water, cook the pasta for 7 minutes. Add the vegetables and cook for 2 minutes or until the pasta is *al dente* and vegetables are tender crisp. Drain well and set aside.

2. Meanwhile, in saucepan heat the oil over a medium heat and cook the onion, thyme and mustard for 2 minutes or until softened. Add the flour and cook stirring for 1 minute. Slowly whisk in the milk, and continue whisking gently for about 5 minutes or until the mixture coats the back of spoon. Remove from heat and stir in the salt and pepper.

3. Add the cooked pasta and vegetables and tuna. Stir to combine well. Scrape into a 23cm (9in) casserole dish and sprinkle with cheese. Bake in a 190°C (375°F; gas mark 5) oven for about 15 minutes or until bubbly and heated through.

Makes 4 servings.

SALMON OPTION: You can substitute 2 cans (213g each) of salmon for the tuna.
CRAB OPTION: You can substitute 200g (7oz) frozen crab, thawed and drained, for the tuna.

SALMON PASTA

For days when you can't get to the market for fresh salmon, use two cans of salmon or tuna instead.

2 tsp rapeseed oil
1 small onion, finely chopped
2 cloves garlic, finely chopped
450ml (16fl oz) chicken or fish stock
115g (4oz) wholemeal macaroni pasta
240g (8oz) chopped broccoli
85g (3oz) light herb and garlic cream cheese
salmon fillet, skinned (about 175g [6oz])
2 tbsp freshly chopped flat leaf parsley
Pinch each salt and freshly ground black pepper

1. In a saucepan, heat 1 tsp of the oil over a medium heat and cook the onion and garlic for about 3 minutes or until softened. Add the chicken stock and bring to the boil. Add the pasta and cover and reduce heat to a simmer and cook for 10 minutes. Stir in the broccoli and cream cheese and remove from heat. Let stand covered for 10 minutes.

2. Meanwhile, rub the remaining oil over the salmon fillet and sprinkle with parsley, salt and pepper. Roast in small baking pan in 210°C (425°F, gas mark 7) oven for about 10 minutes or until the fish flakes easily when tested with fork. Break salmon up into large chunks and add to the pasta mixture. Stir gently to combine.

Makes 2 servings.

FROZEN VEGETABLE OPTION: You can substitute any of your favourite mixed vegetables for the broccoli.

LINGUINE WITH CLAMS 

A staple at most Italian restaurants, this rich-tasting pasta dish is easy enough to make for family dinners and elegant enough to serve at dinner parties.

2 tsp extra virgin olive oil
1 onion, chopped
4 cloves garlic, finely chopped
2 tsp dried oregano
1 tsp dried basil
¼ tsp hot pepper flakes
2 cans (2 x 400g) chopped tomatoes
1 courgette, chopped
2 cans (142g each) baby clams, drained and rinsed
15g (½oz) freshly chopped flat leaf parsley
¼ tsp pepper
Pinch salt
175g (6oz) wholemeal spaghetti or linguine

1. In a saucepan, heat the oil over a medium heat and cook the onion, garlic, oregano, basil and hot pepper flakes for about 5 minutes or until softened. Add the tomatoes and courgette and bring to the boil. Reduce heat and simmer for 10 minutes. Add the clams, parsley, pepper and salt and cook, stirring for about 10 minutes or until thickened.

2. Meanwhile, in large pot of boiling salted water, cook the pasta for about 8 minutes or until *al dente*. Drain and divide among 4 plates. Top the pasta with clam sauce.

Makes 4 servings.

WHITE CLAM SAUCE OPTION: Omit the tomatoes and increase the oil to 1 tbsp; cook the onion, garlic, oregano, basil and hot pepper flakes as above. Add 2 tbsp wholemeal flour and cook, stirring for 1 minute. Whisk in 350ml (12fl oz) skimmed milk and cook, whisking for about 3 minutes or until thickened. Add the courgette, clams and parsley and cook, stirring for 5 minutes. Add the pepper and ¼ tsp salt. Toss with cooked pasta.

POULTRY

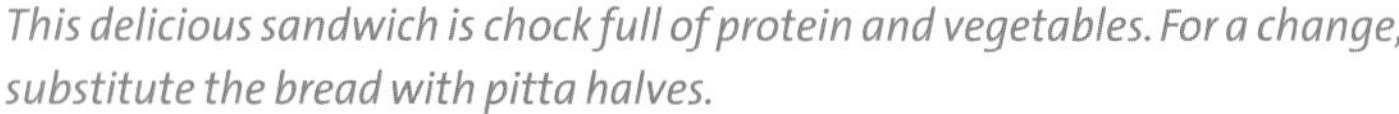

OPEN FACE LUNCH SANDWICH

This delicious sandwich is chock full of protein and vegetables. For a change, substitute the bread with pitta halves.

4 slices stone ground wholemeal bread
½ ripe avocado, peeled and stoned
115g (4oz) cooked chickpeas, chopped
55g (2oz) Light Boursin or Laughing Cow Light cheese
2 tbsp freshly chopped basil or flat leaf parsley
¼ tsp each salt and freshly ground black pepper
4 slices lean ham or turkey (optional)
½ cucumber, chopped
1 plum tomato, chopped
30g (1oz) grated carrot
1 tbsp red wine vinegar
¼ tsp dried oregano

1. Place the bread slices in the toaster or under the grill to toast the bread.

2. In a bowl, using a fork, mash the avocado until almost smooth. Add the chickpeas, cheese, parsley and half of the salt and pepper. Divide and spread over the bread. Top with ham or turkey, if using.

3. In a bowl, combine the cucumber, tomato, carrot, vinegar, oregano and remaining salt and pepper. Divide evenly on the bread.

Makes 2 servings.

TUNA OPTION: Omit the ham and add 1 can (120g) tuna to the cucumber mixture to serve on bread or in pitta.

STUFFED PORTOBELLO MUSHROOMS 

These meaty mushrooms are a novel and tasty alternative to stuffed peppers.

1 tsp rapeseed oil
350g (12oz) lean minced turkey or chicken
30g (1oz) wheat bran
1 onion, finely chopped
2 cloves garlic, finely chopped
1 tsp dried oregano
½ tsp dried basil
Pinch hot pepper flakes (optional)
120g (4oz) baby spinach
60g (2oz) chopped roasted red pepper
½ tsp salt
¼ tsp pepper
2 egg whites, whisked
4 portobello mushrooms
2 tbsp grated Parmesan cheese

1. In a non-stick frying pan, heat the oil over a medium–high heat and cook the turkey, breaking it up with the back of a spoon for about 8 minutes or until no longer pink inside. Drain any fat if necessary.

2. Add the onion, garlic, oregano and basil and cook for about 5 minutes or until the onion is softened. Scrape into a bowl and add the spinach, roasted red pepper, salt and pepper. Let cool slightly. Add the bran and egg white and stir to combine.

3. Meanwhile, remove the stems and scrape out with a small spoon the dark gills from the underside of the mushrooms. Place on a greaseproof paper-lined baking sheet. Divide the turkey mixture evenly onto the scraped side of mushrooms. Sprinkle with cheese and bake in a 200°C (400°F, gas mark 6) oven for about 15 minutes or until the mushrooms are tender.

Makes 4 servings.

SUN-DRIED TOMATO OPTION: Omit the roasted red pepper and use 30g (1oz) sun-dried tomatoes, soaked in boiling water and drained. Chop and add to filling.
VEGETARIAN OPTION: Substitute Quorn mince for the minced turkey.
HELPFUL HINT: To clean mushrooms use a damp paper towel rather than washing them so that they don't absorb the water.

CHICKEN FRIED RICE ●

Chinese fried rice is generally high in fat and low in protein and fibre. This low-Gi version is loaded with chicken and colourful vegetables, and won't leave you feeling hungry again soon after eating it.

350ml (12fl oz) chicken stock (low fat, low sodium)
180g (6oz) brown rice
Pinch salt
1 tsp sesame oil
2 boneless skinless chicken breasts, chopped
225g (8oz) mushrooms, sliced
1 spring onion, chopped
1 carrot, chopped
2 sticks celery, sliced
150g (5 ½oz) cooked chickpeas
50ml (2fl oz) light soy sauce
200g (8oz) bean sprouts

1. In a saucepan, bring 275ml (10fl oz) of the chicken stock, rice and salt to boil. Reduce heat the to low, cover and cook for 25 minutes or until the liquid is absorbed. Fluff with fork and set aside.

2. In a large non-stick frying pan, heat the sesame oil over a medium–high heat and cook the chicken and mushrooms for about 8 minutes or until the chicken is no longer pink. Add the spring onions, carrot, celery, chickpeas and cooked rice. Cook, stirring for 2 minutes to combine.

3. Add the remaining chicken stock and soy sauce and cook for 5 minutes. Add the bean sprouts and toss to combine.

Makes 4 servings.

VEGETARIAN FRIED RICE OPTION: Substitute vegetable stock for the chicken stock. Substitute 275g (10oz) chopped extra-firm tofu for the chicken.
EGG OPTION: Omit the chicken and use 4 medium eggs. In a non-stick skillet, heat 1 tsp canola oil over a medium heat and scramble the egg for about 2 minutes or until no longer runny. Add to the rice mixture with bean sprouts.
HELPFUL HINT: You can use 225g (8oz) of leftover cooked rice and 250g (10oz) of leftover cooked chicken.

CHICKEN CHOP SUEY

It's easy to make this perennial Chinese takeout favourite low-Gi. If you prefer, use a can of sliced water chestnuts instead of the bamboo shoots.

450g (1lb) boneless skinless chicken breasts
2 tsp rapeseed oil
180ml (6½fl oz) chicken stock (low fat, low sodium)
2 tbsp light soy sauce
1 tbsp cornflour
4 spring onions, sliced
1 stalk celery, thinly sliced
1 carrot, thinly sliced
450g (1lb) mushrooms, sliced
200g (8oz) bean sprouts
1 can (227 ml) sliced bamboo shoots, drained and rinsed
1 tbsp freshly chopped ginger

1. Thinly slice the chicken crosswise into bite size pieces; set aside.

2. In a large non-stick frying pan or wok, heat half of the oil over a medium–high heat and cook the chicken stirring constantly for about 8 minutes or until no longer pink inside. Remove to a plate.

3. Add the remaining oil to the frying pan and cook the onions, celery, carrot and mushrooms stirring occasionally for about 5 minutes or until the vegetables are tender crisp. Return chicken to frying pan.

4. Meanwhile, in small bowl, whisk together the chicken stock, soy sauce and cornflour. Pour into the frying pan along with bean sprouts, bamboo shoots and ginger and cook, stirring for about 2 minutes or until the sauce is thickened and bubbly.

Makes 4 servings.

TOFU OPTION: Omit the chicken. Use 450g (1lb) thinly sliced extra firm tofu, and toss with 1 tsp toasted sesame oil; sauté quickly. Continue with recipe.

GARLIC LIME CHICKEN 

The addition of lime gives this chicken a tropical flavour. Serve it with roasted veggies to complete the meal.

6 cloves garlic, finely chopped
1 tbsp grated lime rind
3 tbsp lime juice
1 tbsp rapeseed oil
½ tsp chilli powder or to taste
675g (1½lb) boneless skinless chicken thighs
½ tsp each salt and freshly ground black pepper
12 mini new red potatoes or other small waxy potatoes
3 green or orange peppers
2 tbsp freshly chopped coriander or flat leaf parsley

1. In a large shallow dish, whisk together the garlic, lime rind and juice, half of the rapeseed oil, chilli powder, and half each of the salt and pepper. Add the chicken and turn to coat. Cover and refrigerate for 30 minutes.

2. Meanwhile, cut the potatoes in half and place in large bowl. Cut the peppers in half and remove the ribs and seeds. Cut into thick slices and add to the bowl. Toss with the remaining oil, salt and pepper.

3. Remove the chicken from the marinade and place in the centre of a large greaseproof paper-lined baking sheet. Place the potatoes and peppers around the edge of the chicken and roast in a 210° (425°F, gas mark 7) oven for about 35 minutes or until the chicken is no longer pink inside and potatoes are tender.

Makes 4 servings.

OVEN FRIED CHICKEN LEGS 

Everyone loves fried chicken, but surprise, surprise: it's loaded with fat. The good news is that by using crunchy high-fibre cereal and roasting the chicken in the oven, you can have Gi-friendly fried chicken. Enjoy!

100g (3½oz) bran flakes
1 tbsp grated Parmesan cheese
½ tsp Italian herb seasoning
Pinch each salt and freshly ground black pepper
3 tbsp Dijon mustard
10 skinless chicken drumsticks (about 675g [1½lb])

1. Place the bran flakes into a resealable plastic bag and finely crush. Add the Parmesan, Italian herb seasoning, salt and pepper to the bag and shake to combine. Pour the bran mixture onto waxed paper or shallow dish.

2. Spread mustard evenly over the drumsticks and roll into the bran flake mixture. Place on a greaseproof paper-lined baking sheet and bake in a 200°C (400°F, gas mark 6) oven for about 40 minutes or until the chicken is no longer pink.

Makes 4–5 servings.

CHICKEN STRIP OPTION: Substitute 4 boneless skinless chicken breasts for the drumsticks. Cut each breast into 1 cm (½in) thick strips lengthwise, toss with the mustard and coat with the bran mixture. Bake in a 200°C (400°F, gas mark 6) oven for about 15 minutes.
CHICKEN NUGGET OPTION: Substitute 4 boneless skinless chicken breasts for the drumsticks. For nuggets, cut each breast into 2cm (¾in) inch cubes, toss with the mustard and coat with the bran mixture. Bake in a 200°C (400°F, gas mark 6) oven for about 12 minutes.
BUTTERMILK MUSTARD DIPPING SAUCE: In a bowl, whisk together 60ml (2fl oz) buttermilk, 2 tbsp Dijon mustard, 1 tsp sugar substitute and 1 tsp finely chopped chives. Serve with strips or nuggets.
PORK OPTION: You can substitute pork loin for the chicken breasts.
HERB OPTION: Omit the Italian herb seasoning and use any of dried oregano, thyme or basil.

ORANGE CHICKEN WITH NUTS 

Fans of sweet-and-sour dishes will enjoy this orange-flavoured chicken. The almonds add calcium to this Asian-influenced meal.

2 oranges
1 tbsp rapeseed oil
2 boneless skinless chicken breasts, chopped
2 tsp finely chopped fresh ginger
¼ tsp each salt and freshly ground black pepper
2 spring onions, chopped
1 each red and green peppers, chopped
Pinch hot pepper flakes
50ml (2fl oz) chicken stock (low fat, low sodium)
3 tbsp soy sauce
2 tsp cornflour
55g (2oz) sliced almonds, toasted
Basmati rice (see recipe below)

1. Using a rasp or grater, remove 1 tsp of the orange rind and set aside. Cut away orange rind and pith from 1 of the oranges and discard. Chop orange flesh coarsely. Cut the remaining orange in half and squeeze out juice; set aside.

2. In a large non-stick frying pan, or wok, heat half of the oil over a medium–high heat and cook the chicken, ginger and pinch each of salt and pepper for about 6 minutes or until the chicken is no longer pink inside. Remove to a plate.

3. Add the remaining oil to the frying pan and cook the onions, red and green peppers and hot pepper flakes and cook, stirring constantly, for about 6 minutes or until tender crisp.

4. In a small bowl, whisk together the chicken stock, soy sauce, reserved orange rind and juice, cornflour and remaining salt and pepper. Add the chicken, chopped oranges and sauce to the frying pan and cook, stirring, for about 5 minutes or until the sauce is thickened and chicken and vegetables are coated. Sprinkle with almonds and serve with rice.

Makes 2 servings.

COOKED BASMATI RICE: In a small saucepan combine 350ml (12fl oz) water, 120g (4¼oz) basmati rice and a pinch each of salt and pepper; bring to the boil. Reduce heat to low, cover and cook for 10 minutes or until the rice is tender and water is absorbed. Stir in the 2 tbsp freshly chopped flat leaf parsley.
PORK OPTION: You can substitute 1 small pork tenderloin, chopped, for the chicken.
TOFU OPTION: You can substitute 1 packet (350g) extra firm tofu, chopped for the chicken.

TURKEY MEATLOAF

Meatloaf is a lifesaver for most families since it suits almost everyone's tastes. To please the kids and speed up the cooking time, try the mini muffin variation.

1 tsp rapeseed oil
450g (1lb) chopped mushrooms
1 onion, finely chopped
4 cloves garlic, finely chopped
1 tsp dried thyme
¼ tsp each salt and freshly ground black pepper
175ml (6fl oz) low fat pasta sauce
30g (1oz) wheat bran
1 egg
15g (½oz) freshly chopped flat leaf parsley
1 tbsp Worcestershire sauce
675g (1½lb) lean minced turkey or chicken

1. In a non-stick frying pan, heat the oil over a medium heat and cook the mushrooms, onion, garlic, thyme, salt and pepper for about 8 minutes or until softened and liquid evaporates from mushrooms. Scrape into bowl; let cool slightly.

2. Stir in 50ml (2fl oz) of the pasta sauce into the mushroom mixture. Add the bran, egg, parsley and Worcestershire sauce and combine well. Using your hands, mix in the turkey to combine evenly. Pack the mixture into a 20 x 10cm (8 x 4in) loaf tin and spread the remaining pasta sauce evenly on top. Bake in a 180°C (350°F, gas mark 4) oven for about 1 hour or until the meat thermometer registers 71°C (160°F) when inserted in the centre of the meatloaf. Let cool slightly before serving.

Makes 6 servings.

MINI MUFFIN OPTION: Place the turkey mixture into 12 muffin cups and spread with the remaining pasta sauce. Bake for about 35 minutes or until the meat thermometer registers 71°C (160°F) when inserted in the centre of the mini muffin loaves.

MINCED MEAT OPTION: You can substitute extra lean minced beef for the turkey.

PEPPER OPTION: You can substitute 1 large red or green pepper, chopped, for the chopped mushrooms.

RIGATONI WITH MINI MEATBALLS 

For busy families, a little meal pre-planning always helps during the week. This hearty casserole can be made ahead of time and frozen for another day.

225g (8oz) lean minced chicken or turkey
2 tbsp freshly chopped Italian parsley
1 large clove garlic, finely chopped
1 tsp salt
Pinch pepper
1 tbsp extra virgin olive oil
1 onion, chopped
1 small aubergine, chopped
1 courgette, chopped
1 small carrot, finely chopped
1 tbsp dried oregano
2 cans (2 x 200g) plum tomatoes, puréed
75g (2½oz) cooked red kidney beans
325g (11½oz) rigatoni pasta

1. In a bowl, mix together the chicken, parsley, garlic, pinch of the salt and pepper until well combined. Using wet hands, roll 1 heaping teaspoon of the mixture into small meatballs and place on a greaseproof paper-lined baking sheet. Repeat with remaining mixture. Bake in a 180°C (350°F, gas mark 4) oven for about 8 minutes or until no longer pink inside.

2. Meanwhile, in large saucepan heat the oil over a medium–high heat and cook the onion and aubergine for about 8 minutes or until golden and softened. Reduce heat to medium and add the courgette, carrot and oregano and cook stirring for 5 minutes or until softened. Add the puréed tomatoes and remaining salt; bring to the boil. Add the cooked meatballs and beans; reduce heat and simmer for about 30 minutes or until slightly thickened.

3. In a large pot of boiling salted water, cook the rigatoni for about 10 minutes or until *al dente*. Drain and add to the pasta sauce pot and stir to combine. Pour into a shallow casserole dish.

Makes 4–6 servings.

HELPFUL HINT: To make this dish ahead you can pour the mixture into a casserole dish and let it cool for 30 minutes before covering and placing in the refrigerator. It can remain refrigerated for up to 1 day. You can freeze this casserole dish for up to 2 weeks. Let it thaw in the refrigerator before reheating in a 165°C (325°F, gas mark 3) oven for about 45 minutes or until bubbly; when a knife is inserted into the centre, it should come out hot.
TIP: Purée plum tomatoes in a blender or food processor.

MEAT

LEAN CHUNKY BEEF CHILLI ●

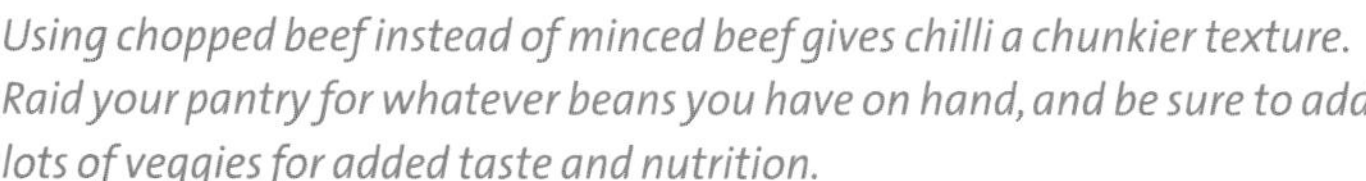

Using chopped beef instead of minced beef gives chilli a chunkier texture. Raid your pantry for whatever beans you have on hand, and be sure to add lots of veggies for added taste and nutrition.

900g (2lb) eye round or
top round of beef
2 tsp rapeseed oil
1 large onion, chopped
3 cloves garlic, finely chopped
1 stalk celery, chopped
1 carrot, chopped
450g (1lb) sliced mushrooms
1 tsp chilli powder
1 tbsp dried oregano
2 tsp ground cumin
1 can (400g) chopped tomatoes
350ml (12fl oz) beef stock
50ml (2fl oz) tomato paste
1 can (410g) chickpeas, drained and rinsed
1 can (410g) red kidney beans, drained and rinsed

1. Cut the beef into 1cm (½in) thick slices. Cut each slice into 1cm (½in) strips then into 1cm (½in) cubes.

2. In a large shallow saucepan, heat half of the oil over a medium–high heat and brown the meat in batches, adding more of the oil as necessary; remove to a plate. Add the onion, garlic, celery, carrot, mushrooms, chilli powder, oregano and cumin and cook stirring for about 10 minutes or until the vegetables are softened.

3. Add the tomatoes, stock and tomato paste and bring to the boil. Add the beef and simmer for about 45 minutes or until the beef is tender. Add the chickpeas and kidney beans; cover and cook for about 15 minutes or until thickened.

Makes 6–8 servings.

MINCED MEAT OPTION: You can also substitute extra lean minced beef, veal, turkey or chicken for the beef.

OPEN-FACED MEATBALL SUBS 

Here's a sandwich hearty enough for dinner. The meatballs can be made with beef, turkey or chicken.

340g (12oz) extra lean minced beef
16g (½oz) wheat bran
15g (½oz) freshly chopped flat leaf parsley
1 egg
1 clove garlic, finely chopped
¼ tsp each salt and freshly ground black pepper
1 jar (700ml) low fat chunky vegetable pasta sauce (tomato based)
1 tsp rapeseed oil
225g (8oz) mushrooms, thinly sliced
1 green pepper, chopped (optional)
½ tsp dried oregano
2 wholemeal submarine rolls, halved lengthwise
70g (2½oz) shredded Cos lettuce
55g (2oz) shredded light style mozzarella

1. In a large bowl, mix together the beef, bran, parsley, egg, garlic, salt and pepper. Using your hands, form the beef mixture into 2.5 cm (1in) meatballs and place on a greaseproof paper- or foil-lined baking sheet and bake in a 180°C (350°F, gas mark 4) oven for about 15 minutes.

2. Meanwhile, in non-stick frying pan, heat the oil over a medium–high heat and cook the mushrooms, pepper and oregano for about 8 minutes or until golden and liquid evaporates from mushrooms. Remove to a plate.

3. Add the pasta sauce to the same frying pan and heat over medium heat. Add the cooked meatballs and bring to simmer. Cook, stirring occasionally, for about 5 minutes or until the meatballs are well coated.

4. Hollow out the inside of rolls leaving 5mm (¼in) around the edge. Divide the lettuce, cheese, mushrooms and pepper mixture among submarine rolls. Top with the meatballs and sauce and serve.

Makes 4 servings.

TOFU OPTION: You can freeze the meatballs after cooking and cooling; after thawing, reheat them in the sauce for a quick evening meal.
HELPFUL HINT: These meatballs can also be eaten without the roll, with the peppers and mushrooms and pasta sauce.

HAMBURGERS FOR EVERYONE 

Make these burgers year-round either on your grill or in a frying pan. Remember to use only half a roll per serving. To make your burgers even more green-light, forget the roll and serve the patties with vegetables.

1 small onion, finely chopped
2 cloves garlic, finely chopped
½ small stalk celery, finely chopped
30g (1oz) fresh wholemeal breadcrumbs
1 egg
1 tbsp Dijon mustard
2 tsp Worcestershire sauce
Pinch each salt and freshly ground black pepper
450g (1lb) extra lean minced beef

Quick Coleslaw
340g (12oz) shredded coleslaw mix
2 tbsp white wine vinegar
2 tsp rapeseed oil
½ tsp celery seed
¼ tsp salt

2 wholemeal hamburger rolls
1 tomato, sliced

1. In a large bowl, combine the onion, garlic, celery, breadcrumbs, egg, mustard, Worcestershire sauce, salt and pepper. Add the beef and, using your hands, combine well and divide the mixture into 4 equal mounds.

2. Shape each mound into 1 cm (½in) thick hamburger patties and place on a greased grill over medium–high heat and cook, turning once, for about 12 minutes or until they are no longer pink inside.

3. To make the quick coleslaw, combine in a bowl the coleslaw mix, vinegar, oil, celery seed and salt; set aside.

4. Divide the hamburger rolls over 4 plates and top with the hamburgers. Divide the tomato slices over the hamburgers and top with the coleslaw mixture.

Makes 4 servings.

HELPFUL HINT: Coleslaw mix is available in the fresh food aisle, where you find other types of salad in bags. It does not contain any dressing. It is usually a mixture of green and red cabbage with some shredded carrot. If this is unavailable, finely shred about ¼ of a small green cabbage.
FRYING PAN OPTION: To cook the hamburgers in a frying pan or grill pan, cook over medium–high heat the for about 15 minutes, turning once.

FRENCH ONION PORK TENDERLOIN MEDALLIONS 

In this dish, French onion soup is transformed into a rich, flavoursome sauce for pork.

pork tenderloin (about 450g [1lb])
2 tsp freshly chopped rosemary
or ½ tsp dried
¼ tsp each salt and freshly
ground black pepper
2 tsp rapeseed oil
2 large onions, thinly sliced
1 red pepper, thinly sliced
2 cloves garlic, finely chopped
350ml (12fl oz) beef stock
1 tbsp Worcestershire sauce

1. Using a chef's knife, trim all the fat from the tenderloin. Cut the tenderloin into 2.5 cm (1in) medallions and sprinkle with rosemary and half each of the salt and pepper.

2. In a large non-stick frying pan, heat half of the oil over a medium–high heat and brown the pork in batches if necessary. Remove to a plate.

3. Return the frying pan to the heat and add the remaining oil. Cook the onions, stirring for about 8 minutes or until beginning to turn golden. Reduce heat to medium and cook, stirring for about 10 minutes or until very soft and golden. Add the red pepper and garlic and cook for 2 minutes.

4. Add the stock and Worcestershire sauce and remaining salt and pepper. Bring to the boil and boil for 5 minutes or until reduced by half. Return the pork to the frying pan and turn to coat in sauce for about 2 minutes or until just a hint of pink remains in the pork.

Makes 4 servings.

MUSHROOM AND GRAVY PORK CHOPS 

Nothing turns food into comfort food better than gravy. For a change, substitute chicken for pork chops.

1 tsp Italian herb seasoning
½ tsp dried basil
½ tsp each salt and freshly
ground black pepper
4 boneless pork loin chops
2 tsp extra virgin olive oil
1 large onion, thinly sliced
450g (1lb) mushrooms, sliced
1 tbsp freshly chopped or 1 tsp dried thyme
2 tbsp wholemeal flour
225ml (8fl oz) chicken stock (low fat, low sodium)

1. In a small bowl, combine the Italian herb seasoning, dried basil and half each of the salt and pepper. Sprinkle evenly on both sides of pork chops.

2. In a large non-stick frying pan, heat the oil over a medium–high heat and brown the chops on both sides; remove to a plate. Add the onion, mushrooms, thyme and remaining salt and pepper and cook, stirring for about 10 minutes or until softened and golden. Sprinkle with flour and cook, stirring for 1 minute. Pour in the stock and bring to the boil. Boil gently for about 3 minutes or until slightly thickened. Return the pork chops back to frying pan and cook, turning occasionally, for about 5 minutes or until the pork has a hint of pink inside.

Makes 4 servings.

CHICKEN OPTION: You can substitute 4 boneless skinless chicken breasts for the pork chops.
VEAL OPTION: You can substitute 8 thin veal leg cutlets or scallopine for the pork chops.

ROASTED GARLIC PORK TENDERLOIN WITH MIXED BEAN TOSS ●

Roasting pungent garlic magically transforms it into a sweet, rich treat. This recipe can easily be doubled for entertaining.

1 head garlic
1 tbsp Dijon mustard
2 tsp freshly chopped or ½ tsp dried thyme
½ tsp cracked black pepper
2 tsp rapeseed oil
pork tenderloin (about 450g [1lb])

Mixed Bean Toss

1 can (410g) mixed beans, drained and rinsed
3 tbsp freshly chopped basil or flat leaf parsley
4 tsp apple cider vinegar
2 tsp rapeseed oil
Pinch each salt and freshly ground black pepper

1. Wrap the garlic in a small piece of aluminum foil and roast in a 200°C (400°F, gas mark 6) oven for about 35 minutes or until soft when squeezed. Let this cool slightly. Squeeze the garlic into a bowl and mash with a fork to form a paste. Stir in the mustard, thyme and pepper; set aside.

2. In a non-stick frying pan, heat the oil over a medium–high heat and brown the tenderloin on all sides. Remove to a small greaseproof paper-lined baking sheet and spread with the roasted garlic mixture. Roast in a 210°C (425°F, gas mark 7) oven for about 20 minutes or until a hint of pink remains in the pork. Let stand 5 minutes before slicing thinly.

3. For the mixed bean toss, stir together in a bowl the beans, basil, vinegar, oil, salt and pepper until combined. Serve with pork.

Makes 4 servings.

HELPFUL HINT: You can roast a few heads of garlic at a time and refrigerate or freeze them. Warm them in the microwave before squeezing.

SNACKS

SOYBEAN HUMMUS 

There are many variations of hummus, a popular Middle Eastern dip. This one uses green soybeans, also known as edamame. You can find them fresh in the produce department of your supermarket, or frozen.

300g (11oz) shelled soybeans
2 tbsp extra virgin olive oil
2 tbsp lemon juice
2 tbsp water
1 small clove garlic, finely chopped
½ tsp ground cumin
¼ tsp salt
Pinch pepper

1. In a food processor, purée the soybeans, olive oil, lemon juice and water until smooth. Pulse in the garlic, cumin, salt and pepper until combined.

Makes about 450ml (1 pint).

SPICY OPTION: For a spicier version of hummus add ½ tsp Asian chilli paste with garlic.

CHEESE AND NUT SPREAD 

This spread makes a delicious snack, or appetiser for dinner parties. The nuts give it a delightfully crunchy texture. Serve it with carrots, celery sticks, cucumber slices or wholemeal pitta triangles.

225g (8oz) no/low-fat cottage cheese
55g (2oz) light Cheddar cheese, grated
85g (3oz) baby spinach leaves,
finely shredded
2 tbsp carrots, finely chopped
2 tbsp spring onion, finely chopped
1 small clove garlic, finely chopped
2 tsp Dijon mustard
½ tsp dried basil
¼ tsp each salt and freshly ground black pepper
3 tbsp chopped toasted almonds

1. In a bowl, stir together the cottage and Cheddar cheeses, spinach, carrots, spring onion, garlic, mustard, basil, salt and pepper until combined well. Scrape into a serving bowl and sprinkle with almonds. Cover and refrigerate for at least 15 minutes before serving.

Makes 8–12 servings.

TOASTING ALMONDS: Place the almonds on a baking sheet and bake in a 180°C (350°F, gas mark 4) oven for about 8 minutes or until fragrant. Watch them carefully to make sure they don't burn. Remove from the baking sheet and let cool. Chop if necessary.

STORAGE: Cover and refrigerate for up to 2 days. Be sure to stir up the mixture before using.

APPLESAUCE BARS 

Perfect for picnics and lunch boxes, applesauce bars can be made ahead of time and frozen.

140g (5oz) wholemeal flour
30g (1oz) wheat bran
30g (1oz) ground flax
10 tbsp sugar substitute
1 tbsp baking powder
2 tsp cinnamon
½ tsp bicarbonate of soda
½ tsp ground nutmeg
Pinch cloves
Pinch salt
450ml (16fl oz) Homemade Apple and Pear Sauce (see next recipe)
3 eggs, whisked
75ml (3fl oz) rapeseed oil
½ tsp vanilla extract

1. In a large bowl, whisk together the flour, bran, flax, sugar substitute, baking powder, cinnamon, bicarbonate of soda, nutmeg, cloves and salt.

2. In another bowl, whisk together the applesauce, eggs, oil and vanilla extract. Pour over the flour mixture and stir until moistened.

3. Scrape the batter into a greased greaseproof paper-lined 33 x 23cm (13 x 9in) baking pan and bake in a 180°C (350°F, gas mark 4) oven for about 30 minutes or until a cake tester inserted in the centre comes out clean. Let cool completely.

Makes 24 bars.

NUTTY OPTION: You can add 60g (2oz) chopped almonds or pecans to the batter before baking.

HOMEMADE APPLE AND PEAR SAUCE 

Served warm or cold, this variation on applesauce makes a nutritious snack. It also makes a wonderful addition to your kids' lunch boxes.

450g (1lb) cooking apples, cored and quartered
450g (1lb) Williams pears, cored and quartered
125ml (4fl oz) apple juice
5 tbsp sugar substitute
½ tsp ground cinnamon

1. In a large saucepan, combine the apples, pears, pear nectar, sugar substitute and cinnamon; bring to the boil. Cover and reduce heat and simmer for about 10 minutes or until tender. Let cool slightly.

2. Scrape into blender or food processor and purée until smooth.

Makes about 700ml (1¼pt).

HELPFUL HINT: If you like a chunkier texture, simply pulse the mixture to get the desired texture.

REFRIGERATOR RAISIN BRAN MUFFINS 

Not many people have time to make muffins on a weekday morning, but if you already have the batter in the fridge, all you have do is scoop and bake. In just 20 minutes, you can have instant fresh muffins for your morning snack.

120g (4½oz) All Bran cereal
350ml (12fl oz) boiling water
225g (8oz) wholemeal flour
50g (1¾oz) wheat bran
11 tbsp sugar substitute
2 tbsp baking powder
2 tsp cinnamon
½ tsp salt
450ml (16fl oz) skimmed milk
2 eggs
50ml (2fl oz) rapeseed oil
50ml (2fl oz) unsweetened apple purée*
or Homemade Apple and Pear Sauce (see recipe left)
2 tsp grated orange rind
85g (3oz) raisins

1. In a bowl, combine the cereal and boiling water. Let stand for 2 minutes and stir to soften.

2. In a large bowl, whisk together the flour, bran, sugar substitute, baking powder, cinnamon and salt.

3. In another bowl, whisk together the milk, eggs, oil, apple purée and orange rind. Pour over the bran mixture and stir to combine. Pour over the flour mixture and stir until moistened. Add the raisins and stir to combine. Cover and refrigerate for up to 2 days.

4. Gently stir the batter before scooping into desired number of greased or paper-lined muffin tins. Bake in a 200°C (400°F, gas mark 6) oven for about 20 minutes or until golden and firm to the touch.

Makes 24 small or 16 large muffins.

DRIED FRUIT OPTION: You can substitute dried chopped apples, dried cranberries or currants for the raisins.
HELPFUL HINT: Bake only as many muffins as you need over the course of the 3 days so you will always have a fresh batch of muffins.

* For unsweetened purée you can make your own or use 'apple only' baby food.

RHUBARB PEAR MUFFINS 

Though rhubarb is best fresh in the summer, you can buy it frozen all year round and use it to make muffins, cakes and compotes. If you find the rhubarb too tart, simply sweeten it with a sugar substitute.

60g (2oz) All Bran or 100% bran cereal
35g (1¼oz) wheat bran
225ml (8fl oz) buttermilk
115g (4oz) wholemeal flour
7 tbsp sugar substitute
2 tsp baking powder
1 tsp grated lemon rind
¼ tsp bicarbonate of soda
Pinch salt
3 medium eggs, whisked
50ml (2fl oz) rapeseed oil
1½ tsp vanilla extract
1 ripe pear, cored and chopped
180g (6oz) freshly chopped or frozen rhubarb

Streusal Topping
30g (1oz) wholemeal flour
3 tbsp sugar substitute
2 tbsp soft non-hydrogenated margarine
½ tsp cinnamon

1. In a bowl, combine the All Bran and wheat bran. Pour over the buttermilk and stir to combine; let stand for 10 minutes.

2. Meanwhile, mix together the flour, sugar substitute, baking powder, lemon rind, bicarbonate of soda and salt. In another bowl, whisk together the eggs, oil and vanilla extract. Stir into the bran mixture. Pour over the flour mixture and stir to combine. Gently stir in the pear and rhubarb until just combined.

3. Divide batter among 12 greased or paper-lined American-style muffin tins (7cm x 3cm [2¾in x 1⅛in]).

4. For the streusal topping, in a small bowl combine the wholemeal flour, sugar substitute, margarine and cinnamon until crumbly. Sprinkle over the top of the muffin batter and bake in a 200°C (400°F, gas mark 6) oven for about 20 minutes or until golden and firm to the touch.

Makes 12 muffins.

STORAGE: Wrap each muffin individually in plastic wrap and freeze in an airtight container for up to 2 weeks or refrigerate for up to 2 days.

OATMEAL CRANBERRY SCONES 

Enjoy these scones with some cottage cheese and fresh fruit for a morning snack or late-afternoon pick-me-up.

140g (5oz) wholemeal flour
30g (1oz) wheat bran
2 tbsp sugar substitute
2 tsp baking powder
¼ tsp ground nutmeg
Pinch ground cloves
115g (4oz) soft non-hydrogenated margarine
100g (3½oz) large flake oats
55g (2oz) dried cranberries, chopped
75ml (3fl oz) skimmed milk
1 egg, whisked

1. In a bowl, combine the flour, bran, sugar substitute, baking powder, nutmeg and cloves. Using your fingers, rub the margarine into the flour mixture until it resembles coarse crumbs. Using a fork, stir in the oats and currants to combine.

2. In a small bowl, whisk together the 50ml (2fl oz) of the skimmed milk and whisked eggs. Pour over the flour mixture and stir until just moistened. Scrape dough out onto floured surface and pat into a 20cm (8in) round, about 2cm (¾in) thick. Cut into 12 wedges, patting edges to re-form slightly. Place onto a greaseproof paper-lined baking sheet and brush the tops with the remaining milk. Bake in a 210° (425°F, gas mark 7) oven for about 12 minutes or until golden brown.

Makes 12 scones.

STORAGE: Let the scones cool completely and freeze in airtight container for up to 2 weeks. Simply reheat them in the microwave or let thaw at room temperature.

DESSERTS

FROZEN RICOTTA TREAT ●

Ricotta cheese is light in flavour and full of protein. By adding a few other ingredients it makes a tasty treat for a hot night or after dinner.

1 tub (500g) light ricotta cheese
4 tbsp sugar substitute
1 tbsp vanilla
225g (8oz) fresh or frozen wild blueberries
225g (8oz) fresh or frozen strawberries, chopped
225ml (8fl oz) no/low-fat strawberry yogurt with sweetener
1 tbsp freshly chopped mint

1. Defrost the fruit if using frozen berries.

2. In a food processor, purée together the ricotta cheese, sugar substitute and vanilla until smooth. Scrape into bowl and stir in the blueberries and strawberries; set aside.

3. Line a 20 x 10 cm (8 x 4in) loaf pan with plastic wrap and scrape the ricotta mixture into the pan, smoothing the top. Cover with plastic wrap and freeze for about 4 hours or until firm.

4. Cut into 2.5 cm (1in) slices and dollop each slice with yogurt; sprinkle with mint before serving.

Makes 8 servings.

BERRY OPTION: Substitute raspberries or blackberries for the strawberries and blueberries.
CRUNCHY OPTION: Add 25g (1oz) All-Bran for added crunch and fibre.
HELPFUL HINT: You can also enjoy this treat without freezing: simply scoop it into small serving dishes and top with yogurt and mint just before serving.

GELATIN FRUIT DESSERT 

Jiggly gelatin desserts are definitely child-friendly. You can easily add variety by using different kinds of fruit. In the summer, use seasonal berries; in the winter, try chopped apples and navel or mandarin oranges.

125ml (4fl oz) water
1 packet (7g) unflavoured gelatin
225ml (8fl oz) unsweetened cranberry juice
5 tbsp sugar substitute
225ml (8fl oz) no/low-fat plain yogurt
1 can (14oz) sliced peaches, no sugar added, drained
155g (5½oz) red seedless grapes

1. Pour the water into a small saucepan and sprinkle gelatin over the top – let stand for 1 minute. Place over a medium heat and stir until the gelatin is melted. Add the cranberry juice and sugar substitute and stir until combined. Refrigerate for about 1 hour, stirring occasionally or until thickened to the consistency of egg whites. Stir in the yogurt until combined.

2. Meanwhile, chop the peaches coarsely and cut the grapes in half lengthwise. Stir into gelatin mixture. Pour into 250ml (8fl oz) ramekins or into a shallow glass dish and refrigerate for about 2 hours or until firm.

Makes 4 servings.

FRUIT OPTION: You can change the fruit to any of your favourite sorts – simply use about 450g (1lb).

APPLE RASPBERRY COFFEE CAKE 

A piece of this fruit-laden cake makes a delectable light dessert. It can be refrigerated for up to three days.

115g (4oz) wholemeal flour
30g (1oz) wheat bran
7 tbsp sugar substitute
1½ tsp baking powder
½ tsp bicarbonate of soda
¼ tsp cinnamon
¼ tsp ground nutmeg
Pinch salt
125ml (4fl oz) buttermilk
55g (2oz) soft non-hydrogenated margarine, melted and cooled
1 egg, whisked
2 tsp vanilla
225g (8oz) fresh raspberries
1 apple, cored and chopped
Topping
35g (1½oz) jumbo oats
3 tbsp sugar substitute
2 tbsp chopped pecans
1 tbsp soft non-hydrogenated margarine

1. In a large bowl, whisk together the flour, bran, sugar substitute, baking powder and soda, cinnamon, nutmeg and salt; set aside.

2. In another bowl, whisk together the buttermilk, margarine, egg and vanilla. Pour over the flour mixture and stir until moistened. Spread two-thirds of the batter into a greaseproof paper-lined 8 inch baking pan. Toss the raspberries and apple together and sprinkle over batter. Dollop the remaining batter and spread gently with a wet spatula.

3. For the topping, mix together in a bowl the oats, sugar substitute, pecans and margarine until combined. Sprinkle over the top of the cake; press into batter gently. Bake in a 180°C (350°F, gas mark 4) oven for about 30 minutes or until the tester inserted in centre comes out clean.

Makes 9 servings.

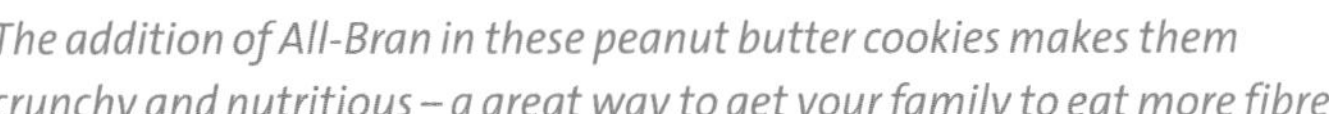

PEANUT BUTTER CRUNCH COOKIES

The addition of All-Bran in these peanut butter cookies makes them crunchy and nutritious – a great way to get your family to eat more fibre.

125g (4½oz) peanut butter (natural, no sugar added)
85g (3oz) soft non-hydrogenated margarine
7 tbsp sugar substitute
1 egg
2 tsp vanilla extract
½ tsp bicarbonate of soda
½ tsp baking powder
Pinch salt
50g (1¾oz) All Bran, crushed
30g (1oz) wholemeal flour

1. In a large bowl, using an electric mixer, beat together the peanut butter and margarine. Add the sugar substitute, egg, vanilla, bicarbonate of soda and powder, and salt, and beat until sticky. Stir in the bran and flour until combined.

2. Scoop out 1 tablespoonful of dough and, using damp hands, roll into a ball. Place on a greaseproof paper-lined baking sheet and repeat with remaining dough, leaving 5 cm (2in) between each cookie. Using a floured fork, flatten cookies slightly with tines of fork.

3. Bake in a 190°C (375°F; gas mark 5) oven for about 10 minutes or until the cookies are light brown on the bottom. Let the cookies cool on a rack for 2 minutes. Remove to a rack to cool completely.

Makes about 18 cookies.

STORAGE: Layer cooled cookies in an airtight container between waxed or parchment paper and freeze for up to 2 weeks, or keep at room temperature for 3 days.

Appendix I

COMPLETE GI DIET FOOD GUIDE

RED

BEANS

Broad

BEANS (TINNED)

Baked beans with pork
Refried beans

YELLOW

GREEN

BEANS

Black
Black eyed
Butter
Chickpeas
Haricot/Navy
Italian
Kidney
Lentils
Lima
Mung
Pigeon
Pinto
Romano
Soy
Split

BEANS (TINNED)

Baked beans (low-fat)
Mixed salad beans
Most varieties
Vegetarian chilli

BEVERAGES

Alcoholic drinks*

Fruit drinks

Milk (whole)

Regular coffee

Regular soft drinks

Sweetened juice

**In Phase II a glass of wine and the occasional beer ma be included see page 99.*

BEVERAGES

Diet soft drinks (caffeinated)

Milk (semi-skimmed)

Red wine*

Regular coffee
(with skimmed milk, no sugar)

Unsweetened fruit juices:

Apple

Cranberry

Grapefruit

Orange

Pear

Pineapple

BEVERAGES

Bottled water

Decaffeinated coffee (with skimmed milk, no sugar)

Diet soft drinks (no caffeine)

Herbal teas

Light instant chocolate

Milk (skimmed)

Tea (with skimmed milk, no sugar)

Soya milk (low-fat, plain)

RED BREADS

Bagels
Baguette/Croissants
Cereal/Granola bars
Crispbreads
Doughnuts
Hamburger buns
Hot dog buns
Kaiser rolls
Melba toast
Muffins
Pancakes/Waffles
Pizza
Stuffing
Tortillas
White bread

YELLOW BREADS

Pitta (wholemeal)
Wholegrain breads
Crispbread with fibre

GREEN BREADS

100% stone-ground wholemeal*
Homemade muffins (see p.227-8)
Homemade waffles (see *p.184*)
Wholegrain, high-fibre breads (2½ to 3g of fibre per slice)*
Crispbreads (high-fibre) *

**Limit portions. See p.25*